T0214898

Anesthesia, Intensive Care and Pain
in Neonates and Children

Series Editors

Antonino Gullo
Marinella Astuto
Ida Salvo

Marinella Astuto

Editor

Pediatric Anesthesia, Intensive Care and Pain: Standardization in Clinical Practice

Foreword by Massimo Antonelli

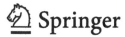 Springer

Editor

Marinella Astuto
Anesthesia and Intensive Care, Pediatric Anesthesia
and Intensive Care Section, and Postgraduate School
University of Catania, AOU Policlinico-Vittorio Emanuele
Catania, Italy

ISSN 2281-1788
ISBN 978-88-470-2684-1   ISBN 978-88-470-2685-8 (eBook)
DOI 10.1007/978-88-470-2685-8
Springer Milan Heidelberg New York Dordrecht London

Library of Congress Control Number: 2012953281

Cover design: eStudio Calamar S.L.
Typesetting: C & G di Cerri e Galassi, Cremona, Italy
Printing and binding: Arti Grafiche Nidasio S.r.l., Assago (MI), Italy

Springer-Verlag Italia S.r.l., Via Decembrio 28, 20137 Milan, Italy

Springer is a part of Springer Science+Business Media (www.springer.com)

To my nephews and nieces

Foreword

This new volume in the series *Anesthesia, Intensive Care and Pain in Neonates and Children* represents a good example of continuity and innovation. Key topics in pediatric critical care, anesthesia and analgesia are discussed in the light of recent insights, building upon the established base of knowledge. By documenting the state of the art, this book will be an excellent update for established practitioners and an essential educational tool for clinical anesthesia and intensive care in children and neonates that will greatly benefit anesthesiologists and intensivists in training.

The vast clinical experience of Prof. Marinella Astuto makes her the ideal editor of a work that will inspire standardization and professionalism by carefully analyzing the various aspects of pediatric critical care and anesthesia and addressing significant problems in monitoring and safety, airway management, clinical anaesthesia and the application of special techniques under different circumstances.

I am confident in the success of this new volume, based on the stimulating contributions that it offers from recognized national and international experts, all coordinated by Professor Astuto, whose talent and motivation are exquisitely expressed in this work.

Rome, November 2012

Prof. Massimo Antonelli, MD
Editor in Chief of Intensive Care Medicine
President of the Italian Society of Anesthesiology
and Intensive Care Medicine (SIAARTI)
Professor of Intensive Care and Anesthesiology
Director of General ICU
and Institute of Anesthesiology and Intensive Care
Policlinico Universitario A. Gemelli
Università Cattolica del Sacro Cuore
Rome, Italy

Preface

The tradition continues; my colleague Professor Marinella Astuto is ready to run the second volume on pediatric anesthesia and intensive care in neonates and children. The success of the previous book on the same topic has represented the starting point for a continuing process supporting education and training in clinical anesthesia and intensive care in children.

Professor Marinella Astuto has been engaged professionally in managing anesthesia throughout the 30 years of her career, which has encompassed more than 15,000 surgical procedures on pediatric patients in various specialties. During this time, Professor Astuto has acquired important skills in respect of basic clinical approach, monitoring and safety, airway management, development of clinical anesthesia, special techniques to be applied routinely or in special circumstances during the perioperative period, acute pain management, and the care of oncologic pediatric patients. These skills have benefited countless patients as well as hundreds of anesthesiologists in training.

I am confident that this second book, which builds on the first and updates knowledge, will prove very successful thanks to Professor Astuto's skills and the excellent collaboration of national and international authorities in the field. Professor Astuto has spent her life in anesthesiology; this book reflects the quality of her work. She is to be considered a true physician who combines a mission to establish excellence in clinical anesthesia with competence, integrity, and professionalism, in accordance with the Physician Charter of the American Board of Internal Medicine (ABIM 2002).

Catania, November 2012

Antonino Gullo, MD
Department and School of Anesthesia
and Intensive Care
Catania University Hospital, Catania, Italy

Preface

After the success of my first masterclass in anesthesia, intensive care and pain in neonates and children, held in September 2007 in Catania, and of the book *Basics*, published by Springer-Verlag, Italy on the basis of the contents of the masterclass, we decided to organize a second one. This was again based on anesthesia, intensive care and pain in neonates and children but continued from where the previous masterclass had left off. It was held in November 2012, in Catania, with a selected group of teachers who have since assisted me in publishing this second book, *Pediatric Anesthesia, Intensive Care and Pain: Standardization in Clinical Practice.*

My goal was to produce a useful guide on perioperative medicine, intensive care and pain management in pediatric patients, from the premature neonate to the child. In order to achieve this goal, I contacted well-known full-time anesthesiologists for children from various university hospitals from around the world. It was their first-class expertise in the field of pediatric anesthesia, perioperative medicine and intensive care that made it possible to provide a comprehensive overview of current standards of anesthesia and intensive care in neonates and children, with a view to promoting standardization in clinical practice.

All of the co-authors worked with enthusiasm to finalize the 16 chapters of this book. I think that the results of their work will be useful to all pediatric anesthesiologists and to others who are interested in this fascinating "world".

I would like to thank Prof. A. Gullo for his continuing support and the encouragement that he offered during the planning and development of this exciting but difficult initiative. Finally, I wish to offer many thanks to my family and my friends for their patience and love.

Catania, November 2012   Marinella Astuto

Contents

Contributors

Giuliana Arena Department of Anaesthesia and Intensive Care, Sant'Elia Hospital, Caltanissetta, Italy

Andrew C. Argent Paediatrics and Child Health, University of Cape Town, Paediatric Intensive Care Unit, Red Cross War Memorial Children's Hospital, Cape Town, South Africa

Marinella Astuto Anesthesia and Intensive Care, Pediatric Anesthesia and Intensive Care Section, and Postgraduate School, University of Catania, AOU Policlinico-Vittorio Emanuele, Catania, Italy

Cristina Bella Pediatric Anesthesiology and Intensive Care Unit, SS. Antonio Biagio e Cesare Arrigo Hospital, Alessandria, Italy

Adrian T. Bosenberg Department Anesthesiology and Pain Management, Faculty of Health Sciences, University of Washington, Seattle Children's Hospital, Seattle, USA

Edoardo Calderini Anesthesia and Pediatric Intensive Care Unit, Fondazione IRCCS Ca' Granda, Ospedale Maggiore Policlinico, Milan, Italy

Elena Capello Anesthesiology and Resuscitation, University of Turin, S. Giovanni Battista Hospital, Turin, Italy

Giorgio Conti Pediatric Intensive Care Unit, Department of Emergency and Critical Care, University Hospital "A. Gemelli", Catholic University of Rome, Rome, Italy

Andrew J. Davidson Anesthesia Department, Royal Children's Hospital, Flemington Road, Parkville, Victoria, Australia

Daniele De Luca Pediatric Intensive Care Unit, Department of Emergency and Critical Care, University Hospital "A. Gemelli", Catholic University of Rome, Rome, Italy

Nicola Disma Department of Anesthesia, IRCCS Gaslini Children's Hospital, Genoa, Italy

Maria Adele Figini Department of Anesthesia and Intensive Care Medicine, San Paolo Hospital, Milan, Italy

Alberto Giannini Pediatric Intensive Care Unit Fondazione IRCCS Ca' Granda, Ospedale Maggiore Policlinico, Milan, Italy

Cesare Gregoretti Department of Anesthesiology and Intensive Care, Azienda Ospedaliera CTO-CRF-Maria Adelaide, Turin, Italy

Antonino Gullo Pediatric Anesthesia and Resuscitation Unit, and Postgraduate School, University of Catania, AOU Policlinico-Vittorio Emanuele, Catania, Italy

Concetta Gullo Department of Anesthesia and Intensive Care, Postgraduate School, University of Catania, AOU Policlinico-Vittorio Emanuele, Catania, Italy

Pablo Mauricio Ingelmo First Service of Anesthesia and Intensive Care, San Gerardo Hospital, Monza, Italy

Giorgio Ivani Division of Pediatric Anesthesiology and Intensive Care, Regina Margherita Children's Hospital, Turin, Italy

Per-Arne Lönnqvist Department of Physiology and Pharmacology, Section of Anesthesiology and Intensive Care, The Karolinska Institute, Stockholm, Sweden

Leila Mameli Department of Anesthesia, IRCCS Gaslini Children's Hospital, Genoa, Italy

Girolamo Mattioli Department of Surgery and Pediatrics, University of Genoa and Gaslini Research Institute, Genoa, Italy

Andrea Messeri Pain Management and Palliative Treatment, Meyer Children's Hospital, Florence, Italy

Carmelo Minardi Department of Experimental Medicine, Milano Bicocca University, Monza, Italy

Giovanni Montobbio Anesthesia and Pediatric Intensive Care, IRCCS Gaslini Children's Hospital, Genoa, Italy

Brenda M. Morrow Paediatrics and Child Health, University of Cape Town, Cape Town, South Africa

Valeria Mossetti Division of Pediatric Anesthesiology and Intensive Care, Regina Margherita Children's Hospital, Turin, Italy

Paolo Murabito Department of Anaesthesia and Intensive Care, University Hospital Policlinico–Vittorio Emanuele, Catania, Italy

Marco Piastra Pediatric Intensive Care Unit, Department of Emergency and Critical Care, University Hospital "A. Gemelli", Catholic University of Rome, Rome, Italy

Alessio Pini-Prato Department of Pediatric Surgery, IRCCS Gaslini Children's Hospital, Genoa, Italy

Fabrizio Racca Pediatric Anesthesiology and Intensive Care Unit, SS. Antonio Biagio e Cesare Arrigo Hospital, Alessandria, Italy

Marco Ranieri Anesthesiology and Resuscitation, University of Turin, S. Giovanni Battista Hospital, Turin, Italy

Ida Salvo Anesthesia and Intensive Care Medicine, Children's Hospital V. Buzzi, Milan, Italy

Stefano Scalia Catenacci Emergency Unit, San Gerardo Hospital, Monza, Italy

Noemi Vicchio Division of Pediatric Anesthesiology and Intensive Care, Regina Margherita Children's Hospital, Turin, Italy

Federico Visconti Pediatric Intensive Care Unit, Department of Emergency and Critical Care, University Hospital "A. Gemelli", Catholic University of Rome, Rome, Italy

Andrea Wolfler Anesthesia and Intensive Care Medicine, Children's Hospital V. Buzzi, Milan, Italy

List of Abbreviations

AAP	American Academy of Pediatrics
ABR	Auditory Brain stem Response
ADARPEF	Association Des Anesthésistes Réanimateurs Pédiatriques D'Expression Française
AEP	Auditory Evoked Potential
AGP	a1-Acid GlycoProtein
ANZCA	Australian and New Zealand College of Anaesthetists
APCV	Assist Pressure Control Ventilation
ARDS	Acute Respiratory Distress Syndrome
ARF	Acute Respiratory Failure
ASA	American Society of Anesthesiologists
BAL	Bronchoalveolar Lavage
BB	Bronchial Blocker
BiPAP	Bilevel Positive Airway Pressure
BIS	BiSpectral Index
BPD	BronchoPulmonary Dysplasia
BVM	Bagvalve-Mask
BW	Body Weight
CCM	Critical Care Medicine
CDC	Centers for Disease Control
CDP	Constant Distending Pressure
CHEOPS	Children's Hospital of Eastern Ontario Pain Scale
CHIPPS	Children's and Infants' Postoperative Pain Scale
CI	Confidence Interval
CLT/f	Clearance Total fraction
CLU/f	Clearance Unbound fraction
CMD	Congenital Muscular Dystrophy
CNS	Central Nervous System
CPAP	Continuous Positive Airway Pressure
CPIS	Clinical Pulmonary Infection Score
CSF	CerebroSpinal Fluid
CSI	Cerebral State Index

CSS	Closed-System Suctioning
CYP	Cytochrome P
DCO_2	CO_2 Diffusion Coefficient
DLTs	Double-Lumen Tubes
DSM	Diagnostic and Statistical Manual of Mental Disorders
DVT	Deep Vein Thrombosis Prophylaxis
EA	Emergence Agitation
ECG	Electrocardiography
ED	Emergence Delirium
EEG	ElecreoEncephalograph
ELBW	Extremely Low Birth Weight
EMLA	Eutectic Mixture of Local Anesthetics
ENT	Ear Nose and Throat
ETA	Endotracheal Aspiration
ETT	EndoTracheal Tube
FEAPA	Federation of European Associations of Paediatric Anaesthesia
FiO_2	Fraction of Inspired Oxygen
FLACC	Face, Legs, Activity, Cry and Consolability
Fr	French size
FVC	Forced Vital Capacity
GFR	Glomerular Filtration Rate
GOR	Gastroesophageal Reflux
GSD	Glycogen Storage Disorder
hERG	Human Ether-à-go-go Related Gene
HFOV	High-Frequency Oscillatory Ventilation
HIV	Human Immunodeficiency Virus
HSA	Human Serum Albumin
ICU	Intensive Care Unit
ID	Inner Diameter
IgE	Immunoglobulin E
IPPV	Intermittent Positive Pressure Ventilation
IQ	Intelligence Quotient
iRDS	Infant Respiratory Distress Syndrome
IV	IntraVenous
IVH	IntraVentricular Hemorrhage
LA	Local Anesthetics
LBW	Low Birth Weight
LMA	Laryngeal Mask Airway
LRA	LocoRegional Anesthesia
LTMV	Long-Term Mechanical Ventilation
MAC	Minumum Alveolar Concentration
MD	Mean Duration
MDR	Multidrug-Resistant
MI-E	Mechanical Insufflator-Exsufflator
MRI	Magnetic Resonance Imaging

NB-BAL	Nonbronchoscopic Bronchoalveolar Lavage
NCPAP	Noninvasive Continuous Positive Airway Pressure
NEC	Necrotizing EnteroColitis
NICU	Neonatal Intensive Care Unit
NMD	Neuromuscular Disorders
NPO	Nil By Mouth
NPPV	Noninvasive Positive Pressure Ventilation
NRS	Noninvasive Respiratory Support
NSAIDs	NonSteroidal Anti-Inflammatory Drugs
OSAS	Obstructive Sleep Apnea Syndrome
oTv	Oscillatory Tidal Volume
PACU	PostAnesthesia Care Unit
PAED	Pediatric Anesthesia Emergence Delirium
PaO_2	Partial Pressure of Oxygen (in the blood)
PCF	Peak Cough Flow
PDA	Patent Ductus Arteriosus
PEEP	Positive Endexpiratory Pressure
PIM	Pediatric Index of Mortality
PPX	PiPecoloXylidide
PRAN	Pediatric Regional Anesthesia Network
PRISM	Pediatric Risk of Mortality score
PSI	Physiologic Stability Index
PSV	Pressure Support Ventilation
PTSD	Post-Traumatic Stress Disorder
PVL	PeriVentricular Leukomalacia
RCT	Randomized Controlled Trial
RDS	Respiratory Distress Syndrome
REM	Rapid Eye Movement
ROC	Receiver Operator Characteristic
ROP	Retinopathy of Prematurity
RR	Relative Risk
SLV	Single-Lung Ventilation
SMA	Spinal Muscular Atrophy
SpO_2	Oxygen Saturation
T1/2	Terminal half-life
TAP	Transversus Abdominis Plane
TIVA	Total IntraVenous Anesthesia
TPN	Total Parenteral Nutrition
TVs	Tidal volumes
URTI	Upper Respiratory Tract Infection
V/Q	Ventilation/Perfusion
VAP	Ventilator-Associated Pneumonia
VCUG	Voiding Cystourethrograms
VLBW	Very Low Birth Weight
Vss	Volume of distribution at Steady State

VTV	Volume-Targeted Ventilation
WBC	White Blood Cell
WCC	White Cell Count

Part I

Intensive Care

Scoring Systems to Assess Severity of Illness in Pediatric Intensive Care Medicine

1

Andrea Wolfler and Ida Salvo

1.1 Introduction

Critical care medicine (CCM) has been developed during the last 30 years with important improvements in both morbidity and mortality. Clinical and epidemiological research, an improved knowledge of the etiology and physiopathology of several diseases, the availability of powerful drugs with reduced toxicity, and improvements of technologies like ventilators and in techniques such as monitoring of vital signs, all contribute to an improved outcome [1]. For clinical research, the appropriate use of disease definitions, for example, sepsis-related diagnosis and acute respiratory distress syndrome, and the evaluation of patient characteristics and severity on intensive care unit (ICU) admission or during ICU stay were fundamental when comparing patients with similar conditions and severity. Mortality risk scoring systems are integral to the provision of modern intensive care, providing a measure of performance both between and within individual ICUs over time. A valid scoring system must predict mortality accurately while adjusting for case mix and disease severity, but it also requires data capture that is feasible in clinical practice. In adults, CCM severity scores were adopted a long time ago and, subsequently, their use was extended to children. The common pediatric intensive care scores identify physical ICU admission as a crucial event and may use data captured either prior or subsequent to ICU admission, or from a combination of both [2].

Presently, scoring systems such as the Pediatric Risk of Mortality (PRISM) score and the Pediatric Index of Mortality (PIM) are widely used in pediatric ICUs (PICUs) and allow the assessment of the severity of illness and mortality risk adjustment in a heterogeneous group of patients objectively, enabling the conversion of these numbers into a numerical mortality risk based on logistic regression analysis. The purpose of their use varies and may include the comparison of severity of illness between differ-

A. Wolfler (✉)
Anesthesia and Intensive Care Medicine
Children's Hospital V. Buzzi, Milan, Italy
e-mail: andrea.wolfler@icp.mi.it

M. Astuto (ed.) *Pediatric Anesthesia, Intensive Care and Pain: Standardization in Clinical Practice*. Anesthesia, Intensive Care and Pain in Neonates and Children
DOI: 10.1007/978-88-470-2685-8_1, © Springer-Verlag Italia 2013

ent treatment arms in clinical trials and the comparison of quality of care between PI-CUs using standardized (i.e., severity of illness-adjusted) mortality rates [3].

Different kinds of scores are now available: generic indexes of mortality risk adopted for all the children admitted in PICUs like the PRISM or PIM scores, specific severity scores to be adopted for specific groups of children like the Pediatric Trauma Score or the Glasgow Meningococcal Sepsis Prognostic Score. Moreover, different scores evaluating the mortality risk following organ failure have been recently developed, for example, the Pediatric Logistic Organ Dysfunction score. All these scoring system have been developed and carefully validated in tertiary PICUs. In this chapter, we describe the PRISM and PIM families of scores.

1.2 The Scoring System

A scoring system needs to be developed, validated, and then applied. The development of a successful scoring system requires: clear, easily defined, and relevant outcome variables; adherence to well-defined methodological standards; and a specified need. To minimize observation bias, data elements used to create a scoring system should be selected a priori and collected blinded from the outcome [4].

For validation purposes, the most stringent test of a scoring system is external validation or the application of the score to a population other than that from which the score was derived. Internal validation, or validation of the score in the population subset or subsets from which the score was derived, should first be performed, because poor internal validation often predicts a model's failure to be validated externally. The validity of a scoring system is based on how well it does what it has been developed to do: to predict death for those patients who are going to die and survival for those who are going to live. The evaluation of the ability of a scoring system to discriminate between these two populations is described by the area under the curve of the receiver operator characteristic (ROC) curve [5]. Calibration through deciles of risk is evaluated using the Hosmer–Lemeshow goodness-of-fit test [6]. Reliability is the ability of a score to predict mortality accurately in various subgroups of patients. Data reliability testing can be accomplished by one of two methods: intraobserver reliability (data remeasured by the same person or clinician) and interobserver reliability (data remeasured by someone other than the first investigator). Generally, interobserver reliability is preferred [4].

1.3 Pediatric Risk of Mortality

Risk adjustment tools that predict death in PICUs have become established over the past 20 years. The Physiologic Stability Index (PSI), first published in 1984 [7], has been updated twice using data from North American PICUs and renamed first as PRISM and, more recently, as PRISM III [8,9]. PRISM III currently provides

Table 1.1 Variables of the PRISM score [8]

Systolic blood pressure (mmHg)	PaO_2/FiO_2 (mmHg)	Total bilirubin	Age in months
Diastolic blood pressure (mmHg)	$PaCO_2$ (mmHg)	Potassium (mEq/L)	Postoperative status
Heart rate (beat/min)	HCO_3 (mEq/L)	Calcium	Pupillary reactions
Respiratory rate (breaths/min)	Glucose	PT/PTT	Glasgow Coma Scale

FiO_2 fraction of inspired oxygen, HCO_3 bicarbonate, $PaCO_2$ partial pressure of carbon dioxide (in the blood), PaO_2 partial pressure of oxygen (in the blood), *PRISM* Pediatric Risk of Mortality, *PT* prothrombin time, *PTT* partial thromboplastin time

the risk adjustment tool for the United States (US)-based Pediatric Intensive Care Unit Evaluations system, which provides comparative reports to participating units under a licensing arrangement. Various versions of the PRISM family of risk adjustment tools have been used extensively in the USA and to some extent in The Netherlands to inform policy and organizational decisions [9,10].

The PRISM score is a second-generation, physiology-based predictor for PICU patients. It was developed from the PSI to reduce the number of physiological variables required for PICU mortality risk assessment and to obtain an objective weighting of the remaining variables [8]. The PRISM score was derived from data collected in PICUs in the USA between 1980 and 1985 [8]. PRISM points are accrued from abnormalities in physiology occurring during the first 24 h of intensive care admission. Age, operative status, and PRISM score are used to predict the risk of death. Statistical techniques were applied to admission day PSI data from four PICUs (1,415 patients, 116 deaths). The resulting PRISM score consists of 14 routinely measured physiological variables and 23 variable ranges (Table 1.1). The performance of a logistic function estimating PICU mortality risk from the PRISM score, age, and operative status was tested in a different sample from six PICUs (1,227 patients, 105 deaths), each PICU separately, and in diagnostic groups using chi-square goodness-of-fit tests and ROC analysis. In all groups, the number and distribution of survivors and nonsurvivors in adjacent mortality risk intervals were accurately predicted. ROC analysis also demonstrated excellent predictor performance (area index = 0.92 ± 0.02) [8].

PRISM III is a third-generation score; it was derived from data collected in units in the USA in 1993 and 1994 based on a sample of 11,165 admissions to 32 PICUs, representing a wide diversity of organizational and structural characteristics, and was published in 1996 [9]. With this revision, the method of assigning points for abnormalities in physiology was refined and variables that adjust for treatment given before intensive care admission and for five specific diagnoses were added (Table 1.2).

Specifically, the physiological variables and their ranges, as well as diagnostic and other risk variables reflective of mortality risk, were re-evaluated to update and improve the performance of the scoring system. In addition, since minimizing the time period for assessing mortality risk is advantageous for evaluating PICU quality, a 12-h prediction model and a 24-h prediction model were developed. The

Table 1.2 Variables of the PRISM III score [9]

Cardiovascular/neurological vital signs		Acid-base blood gases		Hematology tests
1. Systolic blood pressure	4. Heart rate	1. Acidosis	3. Total CO_2	1. White blood cell count
2. Temperature	5. Mental status	2. pH	4. PaO_2	2. Platelet count
3. Pupillary reflex				3. PT or PTT

Chemistry tests		Other factors		
1. Glucose	3. Potassium	1. Nonoperative CV disease	3. Chromosomal anomaly	5. Acute diabetes
2. Creatinine	4. Blood urea nitrogen	2. Cancer	4. Previous PICU admission	6. Admission from inpatient unit
				7. Pre-ICU CPR
				8. Postoperative

CPR cardiopulmonary resuscitation, *ICU* intensive care unit, *PaO_2* partial pressure of oxygen (in the blood), *PICU* pediatric intensive care unit, *PRISM* Pediatric Risk of Mortality, *PT* prothrombin time, *PTT* partial thromboplastin time

aims were to maximize predictive performance while keeping the number of variables and their ranges to a minimum, using variables that are readily available and clearly definable, while maintaining the assumptions inherent in the PSI and PRISM scoring systems that unmeasured variables are assumed to be normal, and to avoid therapeutic variables that may be unduly influenced by practice patterns [9].

The development of PRISM III resulted in several improvements over the original PRISM scoring system. The variables and the ranges in the PRISM scoring system had been originally selected based on the subjective opinions of physicians who developed the PSI. When the PRISM scoring system was developed from these variables, objectivity was added, but a re-evaluation of the original ranges was not undertaken. In PRISM III, the authors objectively reassessed the predictive power of the physiological variables and their ranges, eliminating some ranges that did not contribute significantly to mortality risk and revising the ranges of the physiological variables that were retained. Although these are important changes, the variables with the greatest importance in outcome prediction are the same in both scoring systems: low systolic blood pressure, altered mental status, and abnormal pupillary reflexes. Moreover, age issues, clear data collection instructions, precise variable definitions, and strict rules for patient inclusion and exclusion were addressed at the outset of this study. While age was included as an explicit variable in the original PRISM score, it was included in the PRISM III score in a logically and clinically more convincing form by using appropriate age-adjusted physiological variable ranges. Subsequent model fit evaluations demonstrated the success of these adjustments. A formal operational method for assessing mental status was also established to account for the frequent use of sedation and for paralysis. Other variables included in the prediction model were better defined, making the scoring system less vulnerable. Other risk factors include operative status, pre-ICU care area, pre-ICU cardiac

Table 1.3 Pediatric index of mortality items [11]

1. Booked admission to ICU after elective surgery, or elective admission to ICU for a procedure such as insertion of a central line or monitoring or review of home ventilation (no = 0, yes = 1)
2. If there is one of these underlying conditions, record the code [number in square brackets]:
   [0] none
   [1] cardiac arrest out of hospital
   [2] severe combined immune deficiency
   [3] leukemia/lymphoma after first induction
   [4] cerebral hemorrhage
   [5] cardiomyopathy or myocarditis
   [6] hypoplastic left-heart syndrome
   [7] HIV infection
   [8] IQ probably < 35, worse than Down syndrome
   [9] a neurodegenerative disorder
3. Response of pupils to bright light (both > 3 mm and both fixed = 1, other = 0, unknown = 0)
4. Base excess in arterial or capillary blood, mmol/L (unknown = 0)
5. PaO_2, mmHg (unknown = 0)
6. FiO_2 at time of PaO_2 if oxygen via ETT or head box (unknown = 0)
7. Systolic blood pressure, mmHg (unknown = 120 mmHg)
8. Mechanical ventilation at any time during the first hour in ICU (no = 0, yes = 1)
9. Outcome of ICU admission (discharged alive from ICU = 0, died in ICU = 1)

Also consider collecting: ICU admission number, age, diagnosis, days in PICU, intubation (no = 0 or yes = 1 = an endotracheal tube *in situ* at any time during ICU admission), gestational age (neonates), Apgar score at 5 min (neonates)

ETT endotracheal tube, *FiO₂* fraction of inspired oxygen, *HIV* human immunodeficiency virus, *ICU* intensive care unit, *IQ* intelligence quotient, *PaO₂* partial pressure of oxygen (in the blood)

massage, and previous ICU admission. The relationship between physiological status, as measured by the PRISM III scoring system, and outcomes was calibrated to a contemporary, well-defined, large reference sample (Table 1.3). The set of 32 PICUs represents about 10% of all PICUs in the USA. These units include a wide diversity of organizational structure and patient mixes. This diversity makes the sample sufficiently representative for most units, enabling the PRISM III scoring system to be used in the comparative assessment of PICU outcomes in essentially all PICUs [9].

Overall, all PRISM III prediction models were accurately calibrated and achieved good discrimination. The PRISM III-24 model with the diagnostic and other risk variables performed best. This result was expected, since PRISM III-24 incorporates more information over longer time periods. However, the other models (PRISM III-12 and PRISM III-24) also performed very well and are suitable for quality assessment. The authors recommend using the PRISM III models with the additional variables since these models may increase applicability to a wider variety of case mix samples. The use of the PRISM III-12 model is appealing for quality assessment since, by shortening the time for data acquisition, it better separates the observation from the treatment period, while the PRISM III-24 model is more accurate for individual patient mortality risk assessment. As expected, PRISM III performed better than PRISM, even when limited to the variables originally included in PRISM [9]. Newer versions of severity-of-illness scores, such as PRISM III, will need revisions and recalibrations to maintain their relevance to contemporary patient populations. PRISM has been widely used internationally and the model accurately discriminates between death and survival.

Nevertheless, there are several problems with PRISM. It is not in the public domain and a license fee has to be paid to use the algorithms. Moreover, because it is calculated from the most abnormal values of 14 variables over a 24-h period, it is very difficult to collect the large amount of information needed to calculate PRISM, and therefore many PICUs do not calculate it routinely [11]. Further, worst-in-24-h scores such as PRISM have two serious methodological problems. First, they appear to be more accurate than they really are: in the units involved in this study, over 40% of deaths occurred in the first 24 h, so there is a danger that the score is really diagnosing death rather than predicting it. Second, worst-in-24-h scores blur the differences between units: a child admitted to a good unit who rapidly recovers will have a score that suggests a mild illness, while the same child who is mismanaged in a bad unit will have a score that suggests severe illness—the 'bad' unit's high mortality will be incorrectly attributed to its having sicker patients than the 'good' unit [11].

1.4   Pediatric Index of Mortality

The alternative to the PRISM family of tools is the PIM scoring system, which was recently updated to PIM2 (Tables 1.3 and 1.4) [11, 12]. PIM and PIM2 use data collected at the time of intensive care admission or the time of first contact with intensive care medical staff. The simplicity of the models makes it easier to collect accurate data routinely on large numbers of intensive care patients.

The PIM was developed by the Australian and New Zealand Pediatric Intensive Care study group from data collected between 1994 and 1996 in seven PICUs in Australia and one in the United Kingdom and was published in 1997 [11].

The development of PIM began in 1988 when data from 678 consecutive admissions over 6 months to the PICU at the Royal Children's Hospital in Melbourne, Australia were collected. The variables collected were the 34 PSI variables plus mean arterial pressure, ventilator peak inspiratory pressure (PIP), ventilator positive end-expiratory pressure (PEEP), motor response to pain, immature neutrophil count, total neutrophil count, base excess, and rectal temperature. The worst value of each variable in the first 24 h after admission was recorded for all 678 patients and the admission values were also recorded for the last 230 patients.

Then, in 1990, 814 consecutive admissions were studied. Information was collected at the time of admission and over the first 24 h in PICU about age, gestational age, pupil reaction to light, motor response to pain, base excess, mean arterial pressure, respiratory rate, arterial carbon dioxide tension ($PaCO_2$), PEEP, and PIP. In the third stage of the study, 1,412 consecutive admissions were studied. Information was collected at the time of admission to the PICU and during the first 24 h about all PRISM variables plus information about sex, time in hospital before

Table 1.4 Pediatric index of mortality 2 items [12]

1. Systolic blood pressure, mmHg (unknown = 120 mmHg) 1
2. Pupillary reactions to bright light (> 3 mm and both fixed = 1, other or unknown = 0) 2
3. PaO_2, mmHg (unknown = 0) FiO_2 at the time of PaO_2 if oxygen via ETT or head box (unknown = 0)
4. Base excess in arterial or capillary blood, mmol/L (unknown = 0)
5. Mechanical ventilation at any time during the first hour in ICU (no = 0, yes = 1) 3
6. Elective admission to ICU (no = 0, yes = 1) 4
7. Recovery from surgery or a procedure is the main reason for ICU admission (no = 0, yes = 1) 5
8. Admitted following cardiac bypass (no = 0, yes = 1) 6
9. High-risk diagnosis. Record the number in brackets. If in doubt record 0
   [0] None
   [1] Cardiac arrest preceding ICU admission 7
   [2] Severe combined immune deficiency
   [3] Leukemia or lymphoma after first induction
   [4] Spontaneous cerebral hemorrhage 8
   [5] Cardiomyopathy or myocarditis
   [6] Hypoplastic left-heart syndrome 9
   [7] HIV infection
   [8] Liver failure is the main reason for ICU admission 10
   [9] Neurodegenerative disorder 11
10. Low-risk diagnosis. Record the number in brackets. If in doubt record 0
    [0] None
    [1] Asthma is the main reason for ICU admission
    [2] Bronchiolitis is the main reason for ICU admission 12
    [3] Croup is the main reason for ICU admission
    [4] Obstructive sleep apnea is the main reason for ICU admission 13
    [5] Diabetic ketoacidosis is the main reason for ICU admission

ETT endotracheal tube, *FiO₂* fraction of inspired oxygen, *HIV* human immunodeficiency virus, *ICU* intensive care unit, *PaO₂* partial pressure of oxygen (in the blood)

admission to PICU, need for mechanical ventilation, diagnosis, the presence of a right-to-left cardiac shunt, estimated fraction of inspired oxygen (FiO_2) in unintubated patients, weight, mean blood pressure, each pupil's size and reaction to light, PEEP, PIP, $PaCO_2$, base excess, and plasma sodium. All these variables were analyzed for an association with mortality. Those that were not associated with mortality were then excluded and a preliminary model was developed.

In the fourth stage of the study, information about the variables in the preliminary model (plus plasma sodium and prothrombin time) was collected from consecutive admissions for patients aged less than 16 years to four PICUs in Australia (the learning sample), and one PICU in the United kingdom and three PICUs in Australia (the test sample) (Table 1.4). Each unit collected data from enough consecutive admissions to include at least 20 deaths. The results were good; the model calibrated and showed good discrimination.

PIM2 was developed from data collected between 1997 and 1999 in 13 ICUs, ten in Australia and New Zealand, and three in the United Kingdom. PIM2 was published in 2003 and included 20,787 admissions [12] (Table 1.4). PIM2 was derived from a larger, more recent, and more diverse data set than the one used for the original PIM score. Three variables, all derived from the main reason for ICU admission, were added to the model (admitted for recovery from surgery or a procedure, admitted following cardiac bypass, and low-risk diagnosis). Changes were made to the variable *high-risk diagnosis*: the criteria for cardiac arrest were changed, liver failure was included, and an intelligence quotient below 35 omitted. To test the revised model, the population was divided into a learning and test sample by randomly selecting units, stratified by size of unit and by country. The new model discriminated well between death and survival and calibrated across deciles of risk well.

The authors of PIM claim that the use of data present on admission is better than use of the worst values in the first 12 or 24 h after admission, as it is done when using the PRISM III scoring system. Patients with lower predicted mortality scores on admission who receive *bad* care and deteriorate within the first 24 h will be counted as unexpected deaths if admission scores are used, but will be counted as expected deaths if the most abnormal values in 24 h are used. Those who are against using admission scores argue that values reflecting the physiological status present on admission could reflect a transient state resulting from interventions during transport or in the operating room. To date, no consensus has been reached as to which approach constitutes the gold standard [5].

The use and testing of the PIM2 score in other countries and in different kinds of patients is increasing and the score does not seem to be suitable for all patient typology. A recent study evaluated the PIM2 score in pediatric cardiac surgery patients and the performance was poor, with fair discrimination, and poor calibration and predictive ability; therefore, the authors did not recommend the use in this category [13].

The need to validate a severity score separately in each country appears unquestionable [12] considering the large diversity in structure, organization, staffing, and management among European PICUs [14] with respect to US and Australian ones. Nevertheless, only few studies on validation have been published in the last 10 years and all of them used the PIM2 score, mainly because it is the most recent severity score published for children, it has a free algorithm to calculate mortality risk whereas other scores require a license, and because the small number of variables makes it very simple to collect. Most of these studies reported the experience of single units in Japan [15], Argentina [16], Honk Kong [17] or Croatia [18]: all these four studies demonstrated a good performance of the score. For its characteristics, the score could be considered for developing countries: it is easy to collect, it seems efficient, and it is free [19]. Two studies reported the validation of the score for the entire country with prospective multicenter observational studies: one was made in the United Kingdom in 2006 [20] and one was made in Italy in 2007 [21]. The first presented an assessment and optimization of mortality prediction tools in the United Kingdom through a large, multicenter, nationwide study and showed good discriminatory power but poor calibration for the PIM, PIM2, and PRISM scoring systems. The authors proposed new, United Kingdom-specific coefficients to obtain satisfactory calibration. The second study reported a good calibration and discrimination of the PIM2 score among 18 Italian PICUs. The validity of the PIM2 score might be explained by some intrinsic characteristics that render it less affected by the setting and by the demographic and clinical features of the population admitted to the PICU. One of the main characteristics of this score is that all the variables have to be recorded within the first hour of admission. As a high percentage of deaths occurred in the first 24 h, the PIM2 seems better than other scores requiring 12–24-h data collection [21]. Moreover, due to the increasing use of the saturation level of O_2 in hemoglobin (SaO_2)/FiO_2 ratio instead of the PaO_2/FiO_2 ratio, some authors have published the assessment of the PIM2 score with this new measurement that can be used when blood gas analysis is not available, which is not infrequent in PICUs [22].

The relationship between physiological status and mortality risk may change as new treatment protocols, therapeutic interventions, and monitoring strategies are introduced. Patient populations may also change as new therapies ameliorate the requirement for ICU care, and new patient groups may emerge, often as a result of other medical advances. Predictive models evolve as databases become larger and additional patient characteristics are integrated into the predictive algorithms. Mortality prediction models need to be kept up to date. Changes in referral practices and in the system providing intensive care may change the thresholds for admission to intensive care. Together with changing attitudes to the indications for commencing and discontinuing life support, these factors might potentially alter the relationship between disease and outcome. Further, as experience, and therefore the quantity of data, expand it becomes possible to use a larger and more diverse patient population to develop mortality prediction models [11].

References

1. Epstein D, Brill JE (2005) A history of pediatric critical care medicine. Pediatr Res 58:987-996
2. van Keulen JG, Polderman KH, Gemke RJ (2005) Reliability of PRISM and PIM scores in paediatric intensive Care Arch Dis Child 90:211-214
3. Tibby SM, Taylor D, Festa M et al (2002) A comparison of three scoring systems for mortality risk among retrieved intensive care patients. Arch Dis Child 87:421-425
4. Marcin JP, Pollack MM (2000) Review of the methodologies and applications of scoring systems in neonatal and pediatric intensive care. Pediatr Crit Care Med 1:20-27
5. AG Randolph (1997) Paediatric Index of Mortality (PIM): do we need another paediatric mortality prediction score? Intensive Care Med 23:141-142
6. Hosmer DW, Lemeshow S (2000) Applied logistic regression. John Wiley, New York
7. Yeh TS, Pollack MM, Ruttimann UE et al (1984)Validation of a physiologic stability index for use in critically ill infants and children. Pediatr Res 2:171-179
8. Pollack MM, Ruttimann UE, Getson PR (1988) Pediatric risk of mortality (PRISM) score. Crit Care Med 16:1110-1116
9. Pollack MM, Patel KM, Ruttimann UE (1996) PRISM III: an updated pediatric risk of mortality score. Crit Care Med 24:743-752
10. Gemke RJBJ, Bonsel GJ (1995) Comparative assessment of pediatric intensive care: a national multicenter study. Crit Care Med 23:238-245
11. Shann F, Pearson G, Slater A et al (1997) Paediatric index of mortality (PIM): a mortality prediction model for children in intensive care. Intensive Care Med 23:201-207

12. Slater A, Shann F, Pearson G (2003) PIM2: a revised version of the Paediatric Index of Mortality. Intensive Care Med 29:278-285
13. Czaja AS, Scanlon MC, Kuhn EM et al (2011) Performance of the Pediatric Index of Mortality 2 for pediatric cardiac surgery patients. Pediatr Crit Care Med 12:184-189
14. Nipshagen MD, Polderman KH, De Victor D et al (2002) Pediatric intensive care: result of a European survey. Intensive Care Med 28:1797-1803
15. Imamura T, Nakagawa S, Goldman RD et al (2012) Validation of pediatric index of mortality 2 (PIM2) in a single pediatric intensive care unit in Japan. Intensive Care Med 38:649-654
16. Eulmesekian PG, Pérez A, Minces PG et al (2007) Validation of pediatric index of mortality 2 (PIM2) in a single pediatric intensive care unit of Argentina. Pediatr Crit Care Med 8:54-57
17. Ng DK, Miu TY, Chiu WK et al (2011) Validation of Pediatric Index of Mortality 2 in three pediatric intensive care units in Hong Kong. Indian J Pediatr 78:1491-1494
18. Mestrovic J, Kardum G, Polic B et al (2005) Applicability of the Australian and New Zealand Paediatric Intensive Care Registry diagnostic codes and Paediatric Index of Mortality 2 scoring system in a Croatian paediatric intensive care unit. Eur J Pediatr 164:783-784
19. Garcia PC, Piva JP (2007) Pediatric Index of Mortality 2 (PIM2)—A prognostic tool for developing countries: Easy, efficient, and free! Pediatr Crit Care Med 8:77-78
20. Brady AR, Harrison D, Black S et al (2006) Assessment and optimization of mortality prediction tools for admissions to pediatric intensive care in the United kingdom. Pediatrics 117:e733-742
21. Wolfler A, Silvani P, Musicco M et al (2007) Pediatric Index of Mortality 2 score in Italy: a multicenter, prospective, observational study. Intensive Care Med 33:1407-1413
22. Leteurtre S, Dupré M, Dorkenoo A et al (2011) Assessment of the Pediatric Index of Mortality 2 with the Pao2/Fio2 ratio derived from the Spo2/Fio2 ratio: a prospective pilot study in a French pediatric intensive care unit. Pediatr Crit Care Med 12:e184-186

Diagnosis, Prevention, and Treatment of Ventilator-Associated Pneumonia in Children

2

Brenda M. Morrow and Andrew C. Argent

2.1 Introduction

Ventilator-associated pneumonia (VAP) is usually defined as a nosocomial lower respiratory tract infection occurring in mechanically ventilated patients 48 h or more after initiating ventilatory support. VAP has further been divided into *early-* (≤ 4 days of ventilation) or *late-onset* (> 4 days after starting ventilation) [1]. VAP rates have been variably reported from 2.9/1000 ventilator days in the USA [2] up to 89/1000 ventilator days in India [3]. VAP has been associated with an increased duration of ventilator dependence, pediatric intensive care unit (PICU) and hospital stay, and mortality [4–8], and is accompanied by high financial cost [9,10].

Aspiration may be an important cause of VAP in children. Prolonged mechanical ventilation; genetic syndromes; transport into and out of the PICU; reintubation; prior antibiotic use; continuous enteral feeding; bronchoscopy; transfusion; use of narcotic medication; and immunodeficiency have all been associated with the development of VAP [4,5,7,8]. *Acinetobacter baumannii*, *Escherichia coli*, and *Klebsiella pneumoniae* are the most common organisms isolated from children with VAP in developing countries [6], whereas studies from developed countries have implicated *Pseudomonas aeruginosa*, *Haemophilus influenzae*, *K. pneumoniae*, and *Staphylococcus aureus* as the most common causative organisms [7,8]. Nonbacterial organisms have also been implicated in pediatric VAP, such as yeasts and viruses [6,11].

2.2 Diagnosis

Accurate diagnosis of VAP is important as inappropriate therapy is expensive, may be ineffective, and is associated with the development of antimicrobial resistance

B.M. Morrow (✉)
Paediatrics and Child Health
University of Cape Town, Cape Town, South Africa
e-mail: Brenda.morrow@uct.ac.za

M. Astuto (ed.) *Pediatric Anesthesia, Intensive Care and Pain: Standardization in Clinical Practice*. Anesthesia, Intensive Care and Pain in Neonates and Children
DOI: 10.1007/978-88-470-2685-8_2, © Springer-Verlag Italia 2013

[12]. The precise definition of pediatric VAP according to clinical, pathological, and/or microbacterial criteria is unclear and there is no reasonable gold standard available for diagnosis. To accurately define and identify VAP, clinical changes compatible with pneumonia first need to be observed, proof of lung infection needs to be sought, and the etiological organism identified by means of a highly specific method. Only after clinical improvement in response to appropriate therapy, can one really attribute causality to the identified organisms [13].

2.2.1   Clinical Diagnosis

The most commonly used definitions of VAP are those that have been published by the Centers for Disease Control (CDC) [14], but these are complex and not easily amenable to clinical application. These criteria require at least two serial chest radiographs showing new or progressive infiltrates, consolidation, or cavitation, as well as at least three other clinical signs of temperature instability/fever; an abnormal white cell count (WCC); a change in sputum character or quantity; increased work of breathing, tachypnea or apnea; added sounds on auscultation; brady- or tachycardia; and worsening gaseous exchange. These criteria all have poor specificity relative to pneumonia and/or its etiology and may be highly subjective [15,16]. For example, none of the clinical characteristics, routine laboratory tests, or chest X-rays can accurately differentiate bacterial from viral pneumonia and it is unclear whether leukocyte concentration consistently differentiates between these etiologies. Exposing children to routine radiography to obtain sequential chest X-rays is expensive, may be harmful in terms of radiation exposure, and has not been shown to improve patient management or outcome when compared with restrictive radiography [17].

Using the CDC diagnostic criteria, three independent infection control personnel assessing 50 patients disagreed in almost 40% of the cases and reported a twofold variation in the number of patients with VAP. A kappa score of 0.4 indicated high interobserver variability [18].

The Clinical Pulmonary Infection Score (CPIS) is a clinical tool which rates various clinical and radiographical signs from 0 to 2, with a total score > 6 indicating a high probability of VAP (Table 2.1) [19]. The CPIS has been shown to have poor sensitivity, specificity, and interobserver reliability in adults [20]. However, a simplified CPIS was recently validated against quantitative bronchoscopic bronchoalveolar lavage (BAL) culture in 30 mechanically ventilated children [21] – the mean CPIS was significantly higher in patients with definite VAP, and a CPIS of 8 had a sensitivity and specificity of 80%. These authors suggested that the CPIS is a useful clinical tool to identify children with a high probability of VAP to ensure prompt culture and treatment [21]. Another study of 40 consecutive ventilated pediatric patients reported that the CPIS had a positive predictive value of 93% in the diagnosis of VAP. Furthermore, the CPIS could be considered an early predictor of poor outcome in patients with VAP and also allowed good monitoring of the course of illness [22]. In another study, the sensitivity and

Table 2.1 Clinical Pulmonary Infection Score [24] (the text in *italics* indicates changes made to the simplified CPIS used by Morrow and colleagues [5])

CPIS points criterion	0	1	2
Temperature (°C)	≥ 36.1 and < 38.4	≥ 38.5 and < 38.9	≤ 36 or ≥ 39
	In the case of external cooling give 1 point		
Blood leukocytes (× 10⁹/L)	≥ 4.0 and ≤ 11.0	≤ 3.9 ≥ 11.1 and absence of band forms ≥ 11.1 and ≤ 17.0, no differentiation done	≥ 11.1 and presence of band forms ≥ 17.1, no differentiation done
Tracheal secretions	Absence	Present and nonpurulent (colour: white or light yellow)	Present and purulent (colour: yellow, green, or brown)
Oxygenation (PaO₂) (mmHg)/FiO₂)	> 240 or ARDS *> 240*		< 240 and no ARDS *≤ 240*
Chest X-ray	No infiltrate *OR not done*	Diffuse or patchy infiltrate	Localized infiltrate
Culture of tracheal aspirate (semiquantitative: < 10, 10–100, > 100)	< 10 No previous culture	≥ 10 and ≤ 100	> 100
Organism isolated on NB-BAL	*No or not done*		*Yes*

ARDS acute respiratory distress syndrome, *CPIS* Clinical Pulmonary Infection Score, *NB-BAL* non-bronchoscopic bronchoalveolar lavage, *FiO₂* fraction of inspired oxygen, *PaO₂* partial pressure of oxygen (in the blood)

specificity for VAP diagnosis of a simplified CPIS (Table 2.1) in pediatric patients was found to be high at 100% and 93%, respectively, when compared to the CDC criteria [5]. Advantages of the simplified CPIS (Table 2.1) are that routine radiography and quantitative culture are not necessarily required for the diagnosis of VAP and consideration is given to external cooling as would occur in a servo-controlled environment. The addition of an abnormal procalcitonin (PCT) level to the clinical diagnosis may be useful as PCT is an accurate and early marker of severe bacterial infection in children [23].

2.2.2 Clinical vs. Microbiological Diagnosis of Ventilation-Associated Pneumonia

Blood culture results in childhood pneumonia are frequently negative and therefore not helpful in the diagnosis of VAP, although a positive culture will guide therapy. Routine quantitative endotracheal aspiration (ETA) has been shown to be helpful in guiding antibiotic prescription in adult patients who subsequently developed clinical signs of VAP, which was then confirmed on BAL inspection [25]. However, although negative cultures have a high negative predictive value for VAP, the rate of false positives may also be high, which could lead to the overdiagnosis of pneumonia and result in inappropriate antibiotic use [26]. It is noteworthy that bacterial colony counts compatible with infection were found in up to 80% of ETAs from intubated patients with clinical pneumonia, though they were also found in about 60% of patients without clinical pneumonia, probably as a result of endotracheal tube colonization and biofilm formation [27].

Results from nonbronchoscopic BAL (NB-BAL) are comparable to bronchoscopic lavage and lung biopsy in terms of diagnostic accuracy, with 55–73% sensitivity and 85–96% specificity for the diagnosis of VAP [28]. A comparative study of four diagnostic procedures (ETA, blind bronchial sampling, NB-BAL, and bronchoscopic BAL) showed that NB-BAL was the most reliable sampling method for diagnosing VAP [12]. Clinical criteria were 100% sensitive, but poorly specific (15%) for VAP diagnosis [28]. Combining a sensitive (clinical criteria) and specific (NB-BAL) test may, therefore, achieve good diagnostic validity.

2.3   Prevention of Ventilation-Associated Pneumonia

2.3.1   Infection Control

In the USA, it is estimated that one-third of all nosocomial infections could be prevented by strict adherence to existing infection control policies [29]. Hospital staff have been implicated as a transmission source of nosocomial infections largely as a result of inadequate or poor hand-washing techniques [30]. Therefore, one of the most successful ways of preventing organism transmission is to ensure effective hand washing with soap and water, and regular skin decontamination with alcohol-based solutions [31]. High patient-to-staff ratios significantly impact on the ability of staff to adhere to basic infection control procedures and are associated with a high incidence of VAP [32,33].

2.3.2   Antibiotic Use

Prior antibiotic therapy may select for resistant organisms already present in the respiratory tract, thereby predisposing to VAP. Use of carbapenems and third-generation cephalosporins are independent risk factors for the acquisition of multidrug-resistant *A. baumannii* [31]. Individual PICUs should therefore enforce strict antibiotic restriction policies which specify indications for using carbapenems, cephalosporins, aminoglycosides, vancomycin, and quinolones. The implementation of these policies may be difficult in developing countries where many children are admitted with community acquired infections and are thus on antibiotics from the time of admission. This high primary use of antibiotics may predispose the environment to the development of VAP.

2.3.3   The Bundle Approach

A care bundle approach for the prevention of VAP was developed by the Institute for Healthcare Improvement for adult patients and it has been applied to pediatric practice. The bundle includes: (1) elevation of the head of the bed to between 30° and 45°; (2) daily sedation vacation and daily assessment of readiness to extubate; (3) peptic ulcer prophylaxis; and (4) deep vein thrombosis (DVT) prophylaxis [34]. Additional interventions in children such as closed-system/in-line suctioning, oral hygiene, and oro- rather than nasotracheal intubation, have also been advocated [34].

The premise behind the *bundle* approach to care is that the science behind clinical practice is so well established that it should be considered the standard of care [34]. Implementation of VAP bundles has been associated with a reduction in VAP incidence in adult and pediatric practice, but because of the *all-or-nothing* approach, it is unclear which component(s) are responsible for this improvement.

2.3.3.1 Head-of-Bed Elevation

A randomized controlled trial (RCT) of 86 adult ventilated patients assigned to a supine or 30° semirecumbent position showed that the incidence of VAP was significantly lower in those in the semirecumbent arm of the study, probably as a result of decreased gastroesophageal reflux (GOR) and aspiration [35]. In addition, a semirecumbent position may improve tidal volume and reduce atelectasis [15].

Despite the lack of pediatric evidence to support head-of-bed elevation, it is likely that children and infants have the same, if not greater, risk of GOR and aspiration as adults [34]. Head-of-bed elevation is a low-risk intervention which is likely to hold risks only for patients with specific cardiac disorders or severe sepsis, and is therefore recommended in PICUs. However, logistical difficulties exist in maintaining a minimum 30° elevation, particularly in small children and infants with different body proportions to adults. In infants, a reverse Trendelenburg position has been suggested using bassinets and open incubators [34], but in reality only about a 10–20° inclination is achievable [36]. It is unclear whether such an elevation would be equally beneficial.

2.3.3.2 Daily Sedation Vacation and Daily Assessment of Readiness to Extubate

Prolonged mechanical ventilation is a risk factor for pediatric VAP [4], therefore all available measures to reduce the duration of ventilation should be taken. RCTs in ventilated adults indicate that a *wake up and breathe protocol*, which involves interrupting sedatives and allowing spontaneous breathing, results in reduced duration of mechanical ventilation and ICU stay, and a reduction in mortality, and as such has been recommended as standard practice in adult intensive care practice [37].

Pediatric studies suggest that children are being oversedated in the PICU setting [38] and sedation is known to be associated with increased weaning duration and weaning failure [39]. A 3-year retrospective study showed that children who received neuromuscular blocking agents had longer stays in the PICU, required ventilation for longer periods, and had an increased incidence of VAP [40]. However, *sedation vacations* may not be appropriate for children and infants – the PICU is a foreign and frightening environment for a nonsedated child; inadequate sedation is a risk factor for accidental extubation, while reintubation increases the risk of VAP.

In adults, propofol is frequently used as the sedative of choice, as it allows quick titration of the depth of sedation and also allows rapid emergence on discontinuation of the drug. However, propofol may not be used in pediatric practice, and other narcotics and benzodiazepines lack these titration and emergence characteristics [15]. Therefore, in the PICU setting, it may be preferable to implement a sedation plan to monitor and titrate the level of sedation using scales such as the PICU-specific State Behavioral Scale [41], rather than interrupting sedation on a daily basis. The level of sedation should ideally be such that the child is awake but comfortable and able to breathe spontaneously. Constant heavy sedation should be avoided as this depresses the cough reflex and spontaneous ventilation and predisposes to the aspiration of oropharyngeal secretions [34]. In addition, diaphragmatic inactivity occurring as a result of oversedation may result in rapid disuse atrophy, which could impact on the ability to wean off mechanical ventilation [42].

RCT of 182 infants and children suggested that many patients in the PICU setting need to be extubated and not weaned [39]. In contrast with adult patients, most children are weaned from mechanical ventilator support in 2 days or less and *weaning protocols* do not improve this [39]. Therefore, clinicians should routinely evaluate their ventilated patients' readiness to extubate rather than routinely weaning ventilator support, as routine weaning is likely to prolong the ventilation time of those who were already ready for extubation. Different extubation readiness tests are available [43], with no evidence to support one approach over another.

2.3.3.3 Peptic Ulcer Prophylaxis

Acidification of gastric contents is thought to decrease colonization with potentially pathogenic bacteria. Conversely, neutralizing gastric pH (as would occur when using histamine-2 (H_2)-receptor antagonists and antacids as stress ulcer prophylaxis) may increase colonization, thereby predisposing to VAP. Sucralfate is an alternative agent that does not change gastric pH, therefore it was postulated that it would also decrease the incidence of VAP.

Systematic reviews have suggested that sucralfate therapy is associated with a reduction in VAP and lower mortality compared with H_2 antagonists and antacids in adults [44]. However, a large adult RCT found a significantly greater incidence of stress ulcer bleeding in patients treated with sucralfate compared to ranitidine (an H_2-receptor antagonist) [45]. There was a 15% increase in VAP in the ranitidine group, but this did not reach statistical significance. Therefore, the evidence-based recommendation for adults is to reserve sucralfate for patients at moderate to low risk of gastrointestinal bleeding; and for patients at high risk of severe bleeding to weigh up the potential benefits of sucralfate in preventing VAP against the potential decreased protection against bleeding compared with H_2-receptor antagonists [44].

A retrospective pediatric study of 155 pediatric patients ventilated for > 48 h showed no significant differences in the incidence of VAP between patients treated with sucrulfate or ranitidine [46]. Similarly, a prospective RCT of 160 PICU patients assigned to treatment with ranitidine, omeprazole, sucralfate, or no treatment found no difference in the incidence of VAP, of macroscopic stress ulcer bleeding, or mortality between patients in the different arms of the study [47]. It is not clear whether these studies were sufficiently powered to detect a difference between patients treated with different agents. It is apparent that gastric ulcer prophylaxis is used in the PICU setting [48], and sometimes as part of VAP preventive bundles in children not tolerating enteral feeding [36]. Children who are susceptible to gastric ulceration can receive nonpharmacological gastric protective measures, including early enteral feeding, nasojejunal feeding, and positioning in the semirecumbent position [49].

2.3.3.4 Deep Vein Thrombosis Prophylaxis
DVT prophylaxis is included in the *ventilator bundle* as *excellent practice* [34]. Although it seems sensible to avoid the complication of DVT in sedentary ventilated adults, this practice should not be seen as a VAP-preventive strategy. There is limited data on the risks of DVT in children.

2.3.3.5 Other Interventions

Suctioning System
Some guidelines recommend using in-line or closed-system suctioning (CSS) [34] instead of open endotracheal suctioning, as it was suggested that CSS would reduce the incidence of VAP by eliminating environmental contamination of the catheter before introduction into the endotracheal tube. However, CSS has been found to be associated with significant microbial colonization of the respiratory tract and with bacterial growth on the catheter itself, particularly if the CSS catheter is not changed for extended periods [50,51]. CSS is also less effective at clearing secretions than open suctioning [52].

Meta-analyses of RCTs have found no significant differences between open suctioning and CSS on the incidence of VAP and other outcome measures, including mortality, in adults [51] and neonates [53]. Similarly, a prospective controlled trial of 250 ventilated pediatric patients found no difference in the incidence of VAP or outcome between patients suctioned with closed versus open systems [5]. Therefore, CSS cannot be considered a preventive measure for VAP in any age group.

Oral Hygiene
In adults, dental plaque may become colonized with potentially pathogenic organisms [54], which may predispose to VAP. Meticulous oral hygiene including oral decontamination with chlorhexidine reduces the incidence of VAP in adults [55].

It is unclear how the development of VAP in children relates to the age-related pattern of bacterial colonization connected to the development of dentition [56]. There are no prospective controlled pediatric studies on the effects of oral hygiene on VAP. Recommendations are generally to wipe gums with a gauze in the absence of dentition [34,57], as some commensals can adhere to epithelial surfaces in edentulous infants [56]. Bacterial colonization increases and becomes established after primary dentition emerges, from about 6 months of age, as the teeth provide attachment sites for oral bacteria [56]. Therefore, where teeth are present they should be brushed with toothpaste if possible, and regular oropharyngeal cleaning should be performed with a mouthwash [34,57]. Chlorhexidine has been recommended based on adult data [58]; however, because of its unpleasant taste, a more palatable alternative should perhaps be identified for infants and children.

Orotracheal vs. Nasotracheal Intubation

The link between nosocomial sinusitis and VAP was suggested by a randomized study of 399 nasotracheally intubated adults in whom the incidence of VAP and mortality was significantly lower when sinusitis was actively sought and treated [59]. It has been widely suggested that nasotracheal tubes should be avoided owing to the increased risk of nosocomial sinusitis [34] occurring as a result of blocked paranasal sinus ostia [60]. However, the literature is not clear on this topic – one RCT of 68 ICU patients reported a significantly greater risk of nosocomial sinusitis with nasal rather than oral intubation [61], but another larger RCT of 300 adults showed no significant differences in time to occurrence of nosocomial sinusitis, pneumonia, septicemia, or overall survival rate between the two types of intubation [59]. One cannot therefore conclude that nasotracheal intubation causes nosocomial sinusitis [62].

There are many potential contributing factors to developing sinusitis while in ICU other than nasal intubation. Small diameter tubes such as nasogastric feeding and suction tubes can significantly obstruct the normal flow of sinus fluids, leading to an increased risk of bacterial colonization and the development of nosocomial sinusitis [63]. Heavy sedation is another important risk factor [63] as the normal clearance mechanisms of coughing and sneezing are suppressed [60]. The recumbent position may also increase nasal congestion and cause obstruction of the maxillary sinus ostia [60].

The risk of nosocomial sinusitis in ventilated children and infants has not been assessed, and there is currently insufficient evidence to support oral or nasal methods of intubation in pediatric practice. However, oral intubation carries the risk of airway complications [61]. Conditioned dysphagia has also been reported as a result of multiple medical procedures occurring around the face and mouth [64]. PICU graduates may develop hypersensitivity to touch in these areas and defensive posturing when food is brought to their mouth [64]. In PICUs with staff shortages, consideration should be given to the increased workload needed to prevent accidental extubation of a potentially unstable oral endotracheal tube in minimally sedated patients.

Frequency of Ventilator Circuit Change

Two RCTs ($n = 176$ and $n = 397$, respectively) of pediatric patients assigned to three vs. seven day circuit changes showed no statistical difference in VAP rate between the groups [65,66]. The combined adult literature suggests a reduction in VAP with less frequent circuit changes [67].

2.4   Conclusions and Recommendations

2.4.1   Prevention

Infection control remains the mainstay of VAP prevention, and it is particularly important to emphasize this measure in resource-constrained PICUs with poor staffing levels. Although the *bundle* approach has been shown to reduce the incidence of VAP in adults [34], many components have not been studied in the pediatric age group. In well-resourced countries with sufficient staffing, it may be appropriate to implement a number of low-risk interventions which may have some benefit. However, in developing countries where resources are more limited, any unnecessary interventions should be avoided as this increases the workload of already overloaded nursing staff, predisposing to adverse events [68]. Therefore, to avoid the inappropriate use of scarce resources in an attempt to improve patient outcome, research is needed to evaluate all the *bundle* interventions in the pediatric age group, including efficacy, potential harm, and optimal application.

2.4.2   Treatment

Early effective therapy for VAP is associated with reduced mortality [69]. Therefore, empiric treatment should start promptly on the suspicion of VAP before culture confirmation is obtained. The bacteria causing VAP are increasingly resistant to the antibiotics usually chosen against them [70]. Therefore, initial empiric therapy should use at least two antibiotics targeted at all the likely etiological organisms [71]. Antibiotic therapy should subsequently be rationalized on the basis of culture results [11]. Reverting to a narrow-spectrum antimicrobial agent will reduce the risk of removing commensals and prevent the development of resistance.

On clinical suspicion of VAP, patients should be cultured, preferably from the lower respiratory tract (e.g., by BAL), and empirical therapy changed or discontinued based on these results and on clinical status [4]. Culture results should be considered with other infectious markers such as PCT and band count, and these should be reviewed at 48–72 h. If the cultures are negative and the PCT is low, one may consider stopping the empirical antibiotics unless there are other issues such as immunosuppression or low WCC. An algorithm for the management of VAP, based on adult recommendations, is provided in Fig. 2.1 [72]. We have modified the suggested broad-spectrum antibiotic treatment for suspected multidrug-resistant

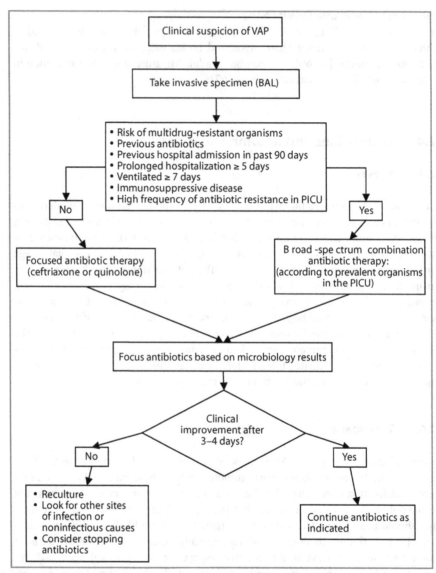

Fig. 2.1 Recommended approach to the treatment of pediatric VAP [13,72]. *BAL* bronchoalveolar lavage, *PICU* pediatric intensive care unit, *VAP* ventilator-associated pneumonia

(MDR) organisms, mainly because of the significant risks for MDR pathogens in PICU settings globally. We are concerned that the use of cephalosporins or β lactam/β lactamase inhibitors or carbapenems in combination with aminoglycosides or fluoroquinolones and vancomycin [72] would predispose to more MDR organisms. It is therefore suggested that unit-based policies should be developed according to the prevalent organisms and resistance profiles in each PICU.

References

1. Hunter JD (2006) Ventilator associated pneumonia. Postgrad Med J 82:172-178
2. National Nosocomial Infections Surveillance System (2004) National Nosocomial Infections Surveillance (NNIS) System Report, data summary from January 1992 through June 2004, issued October 2004. Am J Infect Control 32:470-485
3. Tullu MS, Deshmukh CT, Baveja SM (2000) Bacterial nosocomial pneumonia in Paediatric Intensive Care Unit. J Postgrad Med 46:18-22
4. Foglia E, Meier MD, Elward A (2007) Ventilator-associated pneumonia in neonatal and pediatric intensive care unit patients. Clin Microbiol Rev 20:409-425
5. Morrow BM, Mowzer R, Pitcher R, Argent AC (2011) Investigation into the effect of closed-system suctioning on the frequency of pediatric ventilator-associated pneumonia in a developing country. Pediatr Crit Care Med 13:e25-e32
6. Morrow BM, Argent AC (2009) Ventilator-associated pneumonia in a paediatric intensive care unit in a developing country with high HIV prevalence. J Paediatr Child Health 45:104-111
7. Srinivasan R, Asselin J, Gildengorin G et al (2009) A prospective study of ventilator-associated pneumonia in children. Pediatrics 123:1108-1115
8. Roeleveld PP, Guijt D, Kuijper EJ et al(2011) Ventilator-associated pneumonia in children after cardiac surgery in The Netherlands. Intensive Care Med 37:1656-1663
9. Foglia E, Hollenbeak CS, Fraser V, Elward A (2006) Costs associated with nosocomial bloodstream infections and ventilator-associated pneumonia in pediatric intensive care unit patients. Paper presented at 16th Annual Meeting of Society Healthcare Epidemiology, America. Abstract 109
10. Brilli RJ, Sparling KW, Lake MR et al (2008) The business case for preventing ventilator-associated pneumonia in pediatric intensive care unit patients. Jt Comm J Qual Patient Saf 34:629-638
11. Principi N, Esposito S (2007) Ventilator-associated pneumonia (VAP) in pediatric intensive care units. Pediatr Infect Dis J 26:841-844
12. Sachdev A, Chugh K, Sethi M et al (2010) Diagnosis of ventilator-associated pneumonia in children in resource-limited setting: a comparative study of bronchoscopic and nonbronchoscopic methods. Pediatr Crit Care Med 11:258-266
13. Morrow BM, Argent AC, Jeena PM, Green RJ (2009) Guideline for the diagnosis, prevention and treatment of paediatric ventilator-associated pneumonia. S Afr Med J 99:255-267
14. Horan TC, Andrus M, Dudeck MA (2008) CDC/NHSN surveillance definition of health care-associated infection and criteria for specific types of infections in the acute care setting. Am J Infect Control 36:309-332
15. Wright ML, Romano MJ (2006) Ventilator-associated pneumonia in children. Semin Pediatr Infect Dis 17:58-64
16. Tejerina E, Esteban A, Fernandez-Segoviano P et al (2010) Accuracy of clinical definitions of ventilator-associated pneumonia: comparison with autopsy findings. J Crit Care 25:62-68
17. Graat ME, Stoker J, Vroom MB, Schultz MJ (2005) Can we abandon daily routine chest radiography in intensive care patients? J Intensive Care Med 20:238-246
18. Klompas M (2010) Interobserver variability in ventilator-associated pneumonia surveillance. Am J Infect Control 38:237-239
19. Pieracci FM, Barie PS (2007) Strategies in the prevention and management of ventilator-associated pneumonia. Am Surg 73:419-432
20. Zilberberg MD, Shorr AF (2010) Ventilator-associated pneumonia: the clinical pulmonary infection score as a surrogate for diagnostics and outcome. Clin Infect Dis 51:S131-S135
21. Sachdev A, Chugh A, Sethi M, et al. (2011) Clinical Pulmonary Infection Score to Diagnose Ventilator associated Pneumonia in Children. Indian Pediatr 48:949-954

22. Grasso F, Chidini G, Napolitano L, Calderini E (2004) Ventilator-associated pneumonia in children: evaluation of clinical pulmonary infection score in monitoring the course of illness. Crit Care 8:P209

23. van Rossum AM, Wulkan RW, Oudesluys-Murphy AM (2004) Procalcitonin as an early marker of infection in neonates and children. Lancet Infect Dis 4:620-630

24. Schurink CA, Van Nieuwenhoven CA, Jacobs JA et al (2004) Clinical pulmonary infection score for ventilator-associated pneumonia: accuracy and inter-observer variability. Intensive Care Med 30:217-224

25. Michel F, Franceschini B, Berger P et al (2005) Early antibiotic treatment for BAL-confirmed ventilator-associated pneumonia: a role for routine endotracheal aspirate cultures. Chest 127:589-597

26. El Solh AA, Akinnusi ME, Pineda LA, Mankowski CR (2007) Diagnostic yield of quantitative endotracheal aspirates in patients with severe nursing home-acquired pneumonia. Crit Care 11:R57

27. Jourdain B, Novara A, Joly-Guillou M et al (1995) Role of quantitative cultures of endotracheal aspirates in the diagnosis of nosocomial pneumonia. Am J Respir Crit Care Med 152:241-246

28. Gauvin F, Dassa C, Chaibou M et al (2003) Ventilator-associated pneumonia in intubated children: comparison of different diagnostic methods. Pediatr Crit Care Med 4:437-443

29. Stein F, Trevino R (1994) Nosocomial infections in the pediatric intensive care unit. Pediatr Clin North Am 41:1245-1257

30. Agodi A, Barchitta M, Cipresso R et al (2007) Pseudomonas aeruginosa carriage, colonization, and infection in ICU patients. Intensive Care Med 33:1155-1161

31. Falagas ME, Kopterides P (2006) Risk factors for the isolation of multi-drug-resistant Acinetobacter baumannii and Pseudomonas aeruginosa: a systematic review of the literature. J Hosp Infect 64:7-15

32. Hugonnet S, Chevrolet JC, Pittet D (2007) The effect of workload on infection risk in critically ill patients. Crit Care Med 35:76-81

33. Hugonnet S, Uckay I, Pittet D (2007) Staffing level: a determinant of late-onset ventilator-associated pneumonia. Crit Care 11:R80

34. Curley MA, Schwalenstocker E, Deshpande JK et al (2006) Tailoring the Institute for Health Care Improvement 100,000 Lives Campaign to pediatric settings: the example of ventilator-associated pneumonia. Pediatr Clin North Am 53:1231-1251

35. Drakulovic MB, Torres A, Bauer TT et al (1999) Supine body position as a risk factor for nosocomial pneumonia in mechanically ventilated patients: a randomised trial. Lancet 354:1851-1858

36. Brierley J, Highe L, Hines S, Dixon G (2012) Reducing VAP by instituting a care bundle using improvement methodology in a UK Paediatric Intensive Care Unit. Eur J Pediatr 171:323-330

37. Girard TD, Kress JP, Fuchs BD et al (2008) Efficacy and safety of a paired sedation and ventilator weaning protocol for mechanically ventilated patients in intensive care (Awakening and Breathing Controlled trial): a randomised controlled trial. Lancet 371:126-134

38. Twite MD, Friesen RH (2005) Pediatric sedation outside the operating room: the year in review. Curr Opin Anaesthesiol 18:442-446

39. Randolph AG, Wypij D, Venkataraman ST et al (2002) Effect of mechanical ventilator weaning protocols on respiratory outcomes in infants and children: a randomized controlled trial. JAMA 288:2561-2568

40. Da Silva PS, Neto HM, de Aguiar VE et al (2010) Impact of sustained neuromuscular blockade on outcome of mechanically ventilated children. Pediatr Int 52:438-443

41. Curley MA, Harris SK, Fraser KA et al (2006) State Behavioral Scale: a sedation assessment instrument for infants and young children supported on mechanical ventilation. Pediatr Crit Care Med 7:107-114

42. Levine S, Nguyen T, Taylor N et al (2008) Rapid disuse atrophy of diaphragm fibers in mechanically ventilated humans. N Engl J Med 358:1327-1335

43. Curley MA, Arnold JH, Thompson JE et al (2006) Clinical trial design – effect of prone positioning on clinical outcomes in infants and children with acute respiratory distress syndrome. J Crit Care 21:23-32
44. Collard HR, Saint S, Matthay MA (2003) Prevention of ventilator-associated pneumonia: an evidence-based systematic review. Ann Intern Med 138:494-501
45. Cook D, Guyatt G, Marshall J et al (1998) A comparison of sucralfate and ranitidine for the prevention of upper gastrointestinal bleeding in patients requiring mechanical ventilation. Canadian Critical Care Trials Group. N Engl J Med 338:791-797
46. Lopriore E, Markhorst DG, Gemke RJ (2002) Ventilator-associated pneumonia and upper airway colonisation with Gram negative bacilli: the role of stress ulcer prophylaxis in children. Intensive Care Med 28:763-767
47. Yildizdas D, Yapicioglu H, Yilmaz HL (2002) Occurrence of ventilator-associated pneumonia in mechanically ventilated pediatric intensive care patients during stress ulcer prophylaxis with sucralfate, ranitidine, and omeprazole. J Crit Care 17:240-245
48. Morinec J, Iacaboni J, McNett M (2012) Risk factors and interventions for ventilator-associated pneumonia in pediatric patients. Journal of Pediatric Nursing. In press
49. Turton P (2008) Ventilator-associated pneumonia in paediatric intensive care: a literature review. Nurs Crit Care 13:241-248
50. Freytag CC, Thies FL, Konig W, Welte T (2003) Prolonged application of closed in-line suction catheters increases microbial colonization of the lower respiratory tract and bacterial growth on catheter surface. Infection 31:31-37
51. Jongerden IP, Rovers MM, Grypdonck MH, Bonten MJ (2007) Open and closed endotracheal suction systems in mechanically ventilated intensive care patients: a meta-analysis. Crit Care Med 35:260-270
52. Lasocki S, Lu Q, Sartorius A et al (2006) Open and closed-circuit endotracheal suctioning in acute lung injury: efficiency and effects on gas exchange. Anesthesiology 104:39-47
53. Cordero L, Sananes M, Ayers LW (2000) Comparison of a closed (Trach Care MAC) with an open endotracheal suction system in small premature infants. J Perinatol 20:151-156
54. Munro CL, Grap MJ (2004) Oral health and care in the intensive care unit: state of the science. Am J Crit Care 13:25-33
55. Labeau SO, Van de Vyver K, Brusselaers N et al (2011) Prevention of ventilator-associated pneumonia with oral antiseptics: a systematic review and meta-analysis. Lancet Infect Dis 11:845-854
56. Kononen E (2005) Anaerobes in the upper respiratory tract in infancy. Anaerobe 11:131-136
57. Johnstone L, Spence D, Koziol-McClain J (2010) Oral hygiene care in the pediatric intensive care unit: practice recommendations. Pediatr Nurs 36:85-96
58. Koeman M, van der Ven AJ, Hak E et al (2006) Oral decontamination with chlorhexidine reduces the incidence of ventilator-associated pneumonia. Am J Respir Crit Care Med 173:1348-1355
59. Holzapfel L, Chastang C, Demingeon G et al (1999) A randomized study assessing the systematic search for maxillary sinusitis in nasotracheally mechanically ventilated patients. Influence of nosocomial maxillary sinusitis on the occurrence of ventilator-associated pneumonia. Am J Respir Crit Care Med 159:695-701
60. van Zanten AR, Tjan DH, Polderman KH (2006) Preventing nosocomial sinusitis in the ICU: Comment on article by Pneumatikos et al. Intensive Care Med 32:1451
61. Bach A, Boehrer H, Schmidt H, Geiss HK (1992) Nosocomial sinusitis in ventilated patients. Nasotracheal versus orotracheal intubation. Anaesthesia 47:335-339
62. Stein M, Caplan ES (2005) Nosocomial sinusitis: a unique subset of sinusitis. Curr Opin Infect Dis 18:147-150
63. George DL, Falk PS, Umberto Meduri G et al (1998) Nosocomial sinusitis in patients in the medical intensive care unit: a prospective epidemiological study. Clin Infect Dis 27:463-470

64. Bottei K (1995) Feeding dysfunction: a nursing diagnosis for infants who resist oral feeding. Nurs Diagn 6:80-88
65. Samransamruajkit R, Jirapaiboonsuk S, Siritantiwat S et al (2010) Effect of frequency of ventilator circuit changes (3 vs 7 days) on the rate of ventilator-associated pneumonia in PICU. J Crit Care 25:56-61
66. Hsieh TC, Hsia SH, Wu CT et al (2010) Frequency of ventilator-associated pneumonia with 3-day versus 7-day ventilator circuit changes. Pediatr Neonatol 51:37-43
67. Branson RD (2005) The ventilator circuit and ventilator-associated pneumonia. Respir Care 50:774-785
68. Frey B, Argent A (2004) Safe paediatric intensive care. Part 1: Does more medical care lead to improved outcome? Intensive Care Med 30:1041-1046
69. Luna CM, Aruj P, Niederman MS et al (2006) Appropriateness and delay to initiate therapy in ventilator-associated pneumonia. Eur Respir J 27:158-164
70. Kollef MH (2007) Moving towards real-time antimicrobial management of ventilator-associated pneumonia. Clin Infect Dis 44:388-390
71. Hanberger H, Arman D, Gill H et al (2009) Surveillance of microbial resistance in European Intensive Care Units: a first report from the Care-ICU programme for improved infection control. Intensive Care Med 35:91-100
72. Porzecanski I, Bowton DL (2006) Diagnosis and treatment of ventilator-associated pneumonia. Chest 130:597-604

High-Frequency Oscillatory Ventilation in Intensive Care Units: Children and Neonates

3

Daniele De Luca, Federico Visconti, Marco Piastra and Giorgio Conti

3.1 Introduction

Among unconventional modalities of respiratory support, high-frequency oscillatory ventilation (HFOV) is surely the most commonly used in neonatal and pediatric critical care. Despite it being widely used in the pediatric world, such use is not mirrored in adult critical care and some hospitals and clinics do not use HFOV even for the youngest of patients. This apparent discrepancy is partially due to the lack of strong evidence supporting the benefits of using HFOV in various clinical settings, while gathering significant levels of evidence about some of the associated issues has also proved difficult.

Even when such evidence does exist, the intrinsic characteristics of HFOV make it difficult for many clinicians to understand and therefore to apply the procedure. HFOV is completely different from spontaneous breathing and from any other type of respiratory support. Thus, being so different from the physiology on which respiratory support is usually based, HFOV may be poorly managed. This is one of the main reasons for some of the reported failures in applying HFOV correctly and for the doubts surrounding HFOV.

Nonetheless, HFOV remains a powerful tool for the management of critically ill neonates and children: the purpose of this chapter is to explain the basic mechanical principles of HFOV in a practical way and then briefly review the available evidence for the main indications. Finally, advice about its clinical application will be given.

G. Conti (✉)
Pediatric Intensive Care Unit, Department of Emergency and Critical Care,
University Hospital "A. Gemelli", Catholic University of Rome, Rome, Italy
e-mail: giorgio.conti@rm.unicatt.it

M. Astuto (ed.) *Pediatric Anesthesia, Intensive Care and Pain: Standardization in Clinical Practice*. Anesthesia, Intensive Care and Pain in Neonates and Children
DOI: 10.1007/978-88-470-2685-8_3, © Springer-Verlag Italia 2013

3.2 Basic Principles

3.2.1 Definitions

HFOV is an unconventional form of mechanical ventilation based on the delivery of minimal tidal volumes: since these must be less than the dead space, the term oscillatory tidal volume (oTv) or stroke volume is preferred. Such low oTv is delivered at a supraphysiological rate (usually from 300 to 900 breaths/min). Since the pressure waveform is completely different from the physiological one and has an oscillating shape, synchronization with spontaneous breathing is not possible and again the term oscillation, rather than breaths, should be used. Finally, a third basic aspect of HFOV consists of the *active* expiratory phase. In fact, an oscillatory ventilator will both inject the gas mixture and recover it from the respiratory tree during the pressure oscillation (i.e., during the upward and downward phases of the oscillation, respectively). This active gas movement is typical of HFOV, as other types of respiratory support leave expiration to the elastic recoil forces of the lung tissue. Thus, from a technical point of view, the acronym HFOV may only be used when referring to these specific characteristics. An oscillatory pressure waveform with the same minimal oTv and higher frequencies may be also generated by other systems, without active inflation and deflation: this process is known as nonoscillatory high-frequency ventilation.

3.2.2 Mechanics and Gas Exchange

Due to the characteristics previously described, HFOV may provide efficient and low-stretch ventilation [1], avoiding both overdistension and derecruitment, which should theoretically reduce inflammation and ventilation-induced lung injury [2–6].

Consistently, quite low tidal volumes are currently used in conventional modalities with the same purpose. The low volume excursion is provided by the pressure oscillations, which are so rapid as to not create a significant pressure excursion. In fact, in each instant, the mean airway pressure (Paw) may be considered constant (the so-called constant distending pressure, CDP). This characteristic allows reaching Paw levels far higher than in conventional ventilation, facilitating alveolar recruitment. Conversely, the extremely high frequency and the active gas movement provide a powerful tool to wash out CO_2.

Thus, high CDPs and active expiration are the main determinant of HFOV potency in improving oxygenation and ventilation. These two respiratory functions remain essentially distinct during HFOV, so oxygenation may be improved by increasing pressure and alveolar recruitment, while ventilation strongly depends on oscillation. Therefore, different parameters may almost independently affect lung function.

Nevertheless, gas exchange during HFOV is not completely understood. Since HFOV provides volumes lower than the dead space, mechanisms other than alveolar ventilation should be involved: this nonphysiological characteristic is probably the reason for many misunderstandings about HFOV.

Gas exchange during HFOV has been hypothesized to happen through several mechanisms, such as pendelluft, turbulent flow, radial mixing, Taylor dispersion, and molecular diffusion, among others. Moreover, CO_2 washout in the anatomical dead space is likely to take place. Reviewing such mechanisms is beyond the scope of this chapter. What is important to know is that Eq. 3.1, which is derived from classical physiology studies, does not apply to HFOV:

$$V = (Vt - Vd) \times \text{respiratory rate} \qquad \text{(Eq. 3.1)}$$

(where V is alveolar ventilation, and Vt and Vd are the tidal and the dead space volumes, respectively).

Animal studies [3,7] have demonstrated that ventilation during HFOV is described by a different mathematical model summarized by Eq. 3.2:

$$V = (oTv)^2 \times \text{frequency} \qquad \text{(Eq. 3.2)}$$

(where V is the alveolar ventilation, oTv is the oscillatory volume, i.e., the volume produced by each oscillation, and the frequency (in Hz) is the oscillatory frequency set by the clinician).

Alveolar ventilation during HFOV is usually referred to as the CO_2 diffusion coefficient. This model explains why volumes lower than the dead space are capable of significant ventilation and indicates that the volume produced by the oscillations is more important than oscillation frequency in determining gas exchange (this is shown by the squared value of oTv in Eq. 3.2; see also Table 3.1). Finally, this model confirms that oxygenation and ventilation are separate during HFOV. In fact, while in conventional modalities tidal volume (Tv) will be produced by pressure excursion, in Eq. 3.2 there is no mention of Paw, which is considered to be virtually constant in each instant.

The main determinant for oTv is oscillation amplitude and even more how it is transmitted distally through the airways. The higher the oscillation, the greater the volume produced: thus amplitude (delta P) is the main variable to be set to increase ventilation.

Frequency has a lower impact on ventilation (since it is not squared in Eq. 3.2); however, it has an inverse relationship with oTv, which is more powerful in influencing ventilation. Thus, reducing frequency will not decrease ventilation, because the direct effect of frequency will be easily overcome by the increased oTv^2. Simply,

Table 3.1 Normal values to be considered when using high-frequency oscillatory ventilation in neonates and children [9–11]

	Normal value
oTv	1–3 mL/kg
DCO_2	40–80 $mL^2 \times Hz/kg$

oTv oscillatory tidal volume, *DCO_2* CO_2 diffusion coefficient oTv increases with decreasing frequencies because lower frequencies leave more time for volume generation, provided that the inspiratory time has not been changed; that way, frequency has an opposite effect to what happens during conventional ventilation.

Inspiratory time in HFOV is a variable that is rarely changed and is almost fixed at 33% of the oscillation cycle. Rarely, it has been increased to 50% as a last resource to improve oxygenation, but this may increase the risk of trapping air.

As previously said, the transmission of oscillation across the airways is a main determinant of oTv production. In fact, it is well known that oscillations are dampened while reaching distal airways and this attenuation depends on several factors. First, the diameter of the endotracheal tube is a crucial factor, since the smaller the diameter the greater the attenuation. Second, the ventilator tubing system may significantly attenuate the oscillation if the tubes are soft enough. Similarly, lung compliance affects oscillation transmission and a stiff lung will generally oscillate better than a more compliant one. Oscillation transmission is described by a composite parameter known as oscillatory pressure ratio (OPR), which is the ratio of the oscillation amplitude measured at a given level of the respiratory tree to the delta P set by the clinician. The relationship between OPR and compliance has been described [8] and approaches zero asymptotically with increasing compliance values. These considerations are important because a neonate ventilated with HFOV may have different underlying diseases with distinct mechanical characteristics. The different compliance of patients with acute respiratory distress syndrome (ARDS), bronchopulmonary dysplasia, or pneumonia may differentially affect oscillation transmission and thus ventilation.

Normal values to be considered when using HFOV in neonates and children [9–11] are shown in Table 3.1.

3.3   Evidence-Based Data

There is a significant amount of literature concerning the use of HFOV. It has been widely accepted as a valuable tool to improve gas exchange in infant respiratory distress syndrome (iRDS) and seems to be effective in acute lung injury/ARDS patients. Unfortunately, there is a lack of strong evidence of its usefulness when compared to conventional low-tidal volume ventilation. At first inspection, HFOV appeared an appealing option as a "recruitment strategy". Many animal studies were performed which showed a reduction in lung injury if compared to conventional ventilation, and also a significant improvement in gas exchange [2–6]. Unfortunately, such initial findings were not confirmed by several human trials. For example, in 2006, Marlow and colleagues [12] published a randomized trial with 585 iRDS infants, who were treated with conventional ventilation or HFOV. The patients underwent a 2-year follow-up which showed no significant differences in terms of neurological or respiratory outcomes. In 2006, Soll [13] reviewed the Cochrane meta-analyses and found little clinical benefit using HFOV versus conventional ventilation and stressed the possibility of adverse effects, including the risk for intraventricular hemorrhages and poor neurological development.

In 2009, Henderson-Smart and colleagues [14] analysed two randomized controlled trials (RCTs) involving 199 infants born at or near term (over 34 weeks of gestation). He found no data supporting the use of rescue HFOV in term or near-term infants with severe pulmonary dysfunction. However, he highlighted how neonatal age is complicated by diverse pathologies and by the occurrence of other interventions, which could influence data analysis.

To overcome this problem, in 2010, Cools and colleagues [15] assessed the effectiveness of elective HFOV versus conventional ventilation in pre-term infants. They performed a systematic review and meta-analysis of individual patients' data from 3,229 participants in ten RCTs, with the primary outcomes of death or bronchopulmonary dysplasia at 36 weeks postmenstrual age, death or severe adverse neurological event, or any of these outcomes. This review showed that ventilation strategy did not change the overall treatment effect. HFOV seemed to be as effective as conventional ventilation in pre-term infants, unless it is applied in the early 4 hours of life. In fact, if applied in this early phase of lung injury, HFOV is proved to be able to increase survival of this particular subpopulation.

A well-known role for HFOV is the respiratory management of congenital diaphragmatic hernia associated with pulmonary hypoplasia. In 2007, Migliazza and colleagues [16] described how the early introduction of "gentle" HFOV could affect survival. They reported an overall survival rate of 69%; severity at the onset of HFOV correlated with HFOV failure.

Recent studies suggest a possible role for HFOV after congenital cardiac surgery, despite initial concerns about a potential hemodynamic impairment. In 1991, Meliones and colleagues [17], described how HFOV could be associated with a significant reduction in pulmonary vascular resistance after the Fontan procedure in children.

In 2011, Bojan and colleagues [18] performed a propensity score analysis in a population of infants and children undergoing congenital cardiac surgery; 120 patients were switched to HFOV and matched with 120 controls. The study aimed to assess the short-term outcome in such a population. The length of mechanical ventilation, the length of ICU stay, and mortality rates were compared in the matched set. The results were very interesting: when commenced on the day of surgery in neonates and infants with respiratory distress following cardiac surgery, HFOV was associated with shorter lengths of mechanical ventilation and ICU stay than continuous mandatory ventilation.

Another possible application of HFOV is the treatment of burn patients with inhalation injury. Many ICUs, mainly for adult patients, have a consolidated tradition for the early application of HFOV support for burn patients [19,20]. This technique seems safe and reliable [21,22].

There are some initial experiences of HFOV in children with severe brain injury and concomitant pulmonary disease [23]. Further investigations would be useful to determine the indications and limits of HFOV in such clinical scenarios.

To conclude, HFOV is a valuable tool in the treatment of respiratory distress in the pre-term neonate population. There is no evidence that it can improve outcomes in term or near-term neonates with respiratory distress, if compared to conventional mechanical ventilation. HFOV is considered a rescue therapy for children with ARDS, but there is lack of evidence supporting its role versus conventional low-tidal volume ventilation. Certainly, HFOV is an excellent technique in the "open lung" strategy: it works by improving recruitment in adult patients with severe ARDS [24–26] and acts as protective ventilation, preventing atelectrauma and barotrauma.

Further studies, RCTs, and meta-analyses are needed. However, it seems clear that early application of HFOV in patients with ARDS is more effective [7,24,25,27,28].

3.4 How and When to Use High-Frequency Oscillatory Ventilation

3.4.1 Indications

In this section, we provide some practical suggestions about how and when to use HFOV in pediatric and neonatal critical care (see also Table 3.2). Its use is not scheduled despite many years of experience. However, the following conditions in a neonate have been considered as an elective indication for HFOV:

Table 3.2 List of useful tips driven by the available mechanical and clinical data [36–39]

1. If you think you need HFOV, you will most likely need it: start as early as possible!
2. Use as large a tube as possible.
3. Check perfusion. HFOV uses high mean airway pressure that is supraphysiological just like frequency. This means that higher volume filling and high mean systemic arterial pressure may be needed to oxygenate the patient.
4. Given the low volume excursion, HFOV may facilitate the accumulation of secretions. Check for frequent aspiration. You may use closed aspiration in the more critical phase to avoid derecruitment.
5. Given the low volume provided, active expiration, and the basic mechanics, drug nebulization is not possible during HFOV. Drug delivery is not reliable in such a modality.
6. For similar reasons, the usual measurement of end-tidal CO_2 is not reliable and must not be used. Instead, use transcutaneous blood gas monitoring or insert an arterial line.
7. Use inspiratory times higher than 33% only in the case of failed oxygenation and as a last resource.
8. Uncuff the tube in case of intractable hypercarbia, as a last resource.
9. Do not fear the high mean airway pressure values. The low excursion allows a very low risk of air leaks unlike conventional modalities.
10. Titrate the delta P values with the chest oscillation and CO_2 levels. The ideal delta P value is one that can provide visible chest oscillation and a fair CO_2 decrease.

HFOV high-frequency oscillatory ventilation

- pulmonary hypoplasia;
- CDH;
- meconium aspiration syndrome;
- severe air leaks developed during conventional ventilation.

Rescue HFOV in neonates is often considered when peak or plateau pressures reach values above 25 cm H_2O and/or with intractable hypercarbia, when high levels of FiO_2 are required, irrespectively of the basic diagnosis [11,29,30].

HFOV in children with severe acute respiratory failure is usually considered when the plateau pressure is approaching 30 cm H_2O or when the Paw in conventional modalities is above 15 cm H_2O, despite permissive hypercarbia [31–34]. This has been described for ARDS but also for rare conditions such as status asthmaticus, severe air leaks, and pulmonary hypertension [29], among others. Elective HFOV in the pediatric setting has also been used for perioperative care after cardiac surgery [17,18,35] and for traumatic brain injury [23].

In general, HFOV, both in neonates and children, remains the most powerful rescue tool to avoid extracorporeal life support when conventional measures fail [7,31,32]; to maximize this goal, clearly HFOV should be applied as early as possible [27].

3.4.2 Parameters

HFOV is generally applied at 2–5 cm H_2O of Paw above the level reached in conventional ventilation both for neonates and children. Then, airway pressure must be titrated according to the recruitment maneuvers and the optimal Paw on the deflation limb of the respiratory cycle must be chosen (optimum lung volume strategy). Conversely, the Paw should be set 2–3 cm H_2O below the level in conventional ventilation if HFOV is applied because of severe air leaks: in this case, Paw must be titrated to the minimum level to achieve good oxygenation (minimum lung volume strategy). In this particular case, frequencies higher than the values usually chosen for the size of the patient should be used; this will further minimize flow through any air leaks.

The initial delta P may be 30–40 both for neonates and children and it must be increased until a good chest oscillation and an acceptable CO_2 levels are achieved. Clinicians must be advised that, usually, CO_2 changes quickly during HFOV and that thus the first phases in particular should be closely monitored.

The starting frequency is inversely proportional to the size of the patient: it may be 10–15 Hz for pre-term infants, 8–10 Hz for infants, 5–8 Hz for toddlers and children, and 3–4 Hz for adults. When looking at the size of the patient, the ideal body weight should be considered, unless the baby is a neonate too small for gestational age or an infant with significant failure to thrive.

When facing hypercarbia, the delta P should be increased first, then the frequency should be reduced only if high delta P values have not achieved normocarbia. Please note that reducing the frequency has usually a marked and rapid effect on CO_2, so CO_2 must be monitored to avoid hypocarbia.

References

1. Jane Pillow (2005) High frequency oscillatory ventilation: Mechanisms of gas exchange and lung mechanics. Crit Care Med 33(3 suppl): S135-S141
2. McCulloch PR, Forkert PG, Froese AB (1988) Lung volume maintenance prevents lung injury during high frequency oscillatory ventilation in surfactant-deficient rabbits. Am Rev Respir Dis 137(5):1185-1192
3. Boynton BR, Hammond MD, Freberg JJ et al (1989) Gas exchange in healthy rabbits during high-frequency oscillatory ventilation. J Appl Physiol 66:1343-1351
4. Kamitsuka MD, Boynton BR, Villanueva D et al (1990) Frequency, tidal volume and mean airway pressure combinations that provide adequate gas exchange and low alveolar pressure during high frequency oscillatory ventilation in rabbits. Pediatr Res 27:64
5. von der Hardt K, Kandler MA, Fink L et al (2004) High frequency oscillatory ventilation suppresses inflammatory response in lung tissue and microdissected alveolar macrophages in surfactant depleted piglets. Pediatr Res. Feb 55(2):339-46. Epub 2003 Dec 8
6. Delemos RA, Coalson JJ, Gerstmann DR et al (1987) Ventilatory management of infant baboons with hyaline membrane disease: the use of high frequency ventilation. Pediatr Res 21:594-602
7. Ventre KM, Arnold JH (2004) High frequency oscillatory ventilation in acute respiratory failure. Paediatr Respir Rev 5:323-332
8. van Genderingen HR, Versprille A, Leenhoven T et al (2001) Reduction of oscillatory pressure along the endotracheal tube is indicative for maximal respiratory compliance during high-frequency oscillatory ventilation: a mathematical model study. Pediatr Pulmonol Jun 31(6):458-463
9. Arnold JH, Anas NG, Luckett P et al (2000) High frequency oscillatory ventilation in pediatric respiratory failure: a multicenter experience. Crit Care Med 28:3912-3919
10. Arnold JH, Hanson JH, Toro-Figuero LO et al (1994) Prospective, randomised comparison of high-frequency oscillatory ventilation and conventional mechanical ventilation in pediatric respiratory failure. Crit Care Med 22:1530-1539
11. Froese AB, Kinsella JP (2005) High-frequency oscillatory ventilation: Lessons from the neonatal/pediatric experience. Crit Care Med 33:S115-S121
12. Marlow N, Greenough A, Peacock JL et al (2006) Randomised trial of high frequency oscillatory ventilation or conventional ventilation in babies of gestational age 28 weeks or less: respiratory and neurological outcomes at 2 years. Arch Dis Child Fetal Neonatal Ed 91:F320-F326
13. Soll RF (2006) The clinical impact of high frequency ventilation: review of the Cochrane meta-analyses. J Perinatol 26(Suppl 1):S38-S42
14. Henderson-Smart DJ, De Paoli AG, Clark RH et al (2009) High frequency oscillatory ventilation versus conventional ventilation for infants with severe pulmonary dysfunction born at or near term. Cochrane Database of Systematic Reviews, Issue 3. Art. No.: CD002974
15. Cools F, Askie LM, Off Ringa M, on behalf of the PreVILIG collaboration (2010) Elective high-frequency oscillatory versus conventional ventilation in preterm infants: a systematic review and meta-analysis of individual patients' data Lancet 375:2082-2091
16. Migliazza L, Bellan C, Alberti D et al (2007) Retrospective study of 111 cases of congenital diaphragmatic hernia treated with early high-frequency oscillatory ventilation and presurgical stabilization. J Ped Surg 42:1526-1532
17. Meliones JN, Bove EL, Dekeon MK et al (1991) High-frequency jet ventilation improves cardiac function after the Fontan procedure. Circulation 84:III,364-368
18. Bojan et al (2011) High-frequency oscillatory ventilation and short-term outcome in neonates and infants undergoing cardiac surgery: a propensity score analysis. Critical Care 15:R259
19. Cartotto R, Ellis S, Gomez M et al (2004) High frequency oscillatory ventilation in burn patients with the acute respiratory distress syndrome. Burns 30(5):453-463

20. Cartotto R, Ellis S, Smith T (2005) Use of high-frequency oscillatory ventilation in burn patients. Crit Care Med Mar 33(3 Suppl):S175-S181

21. Walia G, Jada G, Cartotto R (2011) Anesthesia and intraoperative high-frequency oscillatory ventilation during burn surgery. J Burn Care Res 32(1):118-123

22. Cioffi WG, de Lemos RA, Coalson JJ et al (1993) Decreased pulmonary damage in primates with inhalation injury treated with high-frequency ventilation. Ann Surg. Sep 218(3):328-35; discussion 335-337

23. Lo TY, Jones PA, Freeman JA et al (2008) The role of high frequency oscillatory ventilation in the management of children with severe traumatic brain injury and concomitant lung pathology. Pediatr Crit Care Med Sep 9(5):e38-e42

24. Finkielman JD, Gajic O, Farmer JC et al (2006) The initial Mayo Clinic experience using high-frequency oscillatory ventilation for adult patients: a retrospective study. BMC Emerg Med 6:2

25. Mehta S, Granton J, MacDonald RJ et al (2004) High-frequency oscillatory ventilation in adults: the Toronto experience. Chest 126:518-527

26. Wunsch H, Mapstone J, Takala J (2005) High-frequency ventilation versus conventional ventilation for the treatment of acute lung injury and acute respiratory distress syndrome: a systematic review and cochrane analyses. Anesth Analg Jun 100(6):1765-1772

27. De Luca D, Piastra M, Conti G (2011) Kinetics of oxygenation improvement and the timing of HFOV institution. Pediatr Pulmonol Dec 46(12):1251-1252

28. Fedora M, Klimovic M, Seda M et al (2000) Effect of early intervention of high-frequency oscillatory ventilation on the outcome in pediatric acute respiratory distress syndrome. Bratisl Lek Listy 101(1):8-13

29. Kohelet C, Perlman M, Kirpalani H et al (1998) High-frequency oscillation in the rescue of infants with persistent pulmonary hypertension. Crit Care Med 16:510-516

30. Berner ME, Hanquinet S, Rimensberger PC (2008) High frequency oscillatory ventilation for respiratory failure due to RSV bronchiolitis. Intensive Care Med 34(9):1698-702. Epub 2008 May 24

31. Ben Jaballah N, Khaldi A, Mnif K et al (2006) High-frequency oscillatory ventilation in pediatric patients with acute respiratory failure. Pediatr Crit Care Med 7:362-367

32. Clark RH, Yoder BA, Sell MS (1994) Prospective, randomized comparison of high-frequency oscillation and conventional ventilation in candidates for extracorporeal membrane oxygenation. J Pediatr 124:447-454

33. Ten IS, Anderson MR (2006) Is high-frequency ventilation more beneficial than low-tidal volume conventional ventilation? Respir Care Clin N Am 12(3):437-451

34. Rotta AT, Steinhorn DM (2006) Is permissive hypercapnia a beneficial strategy for pediatric acute lung injury? Respir Care Clin N Am 12(3):371-387

35. Kneyber MC (2011) High-frequency oscillatory ventilation and pediatric cardiac surgery: Yes, we can! Crit Care 15(6):1011. Epub 2011 Nov 24

36. Slee-Wijffels FYAM, van der Vaart KRM, Twisk JWR et al (2005) High Frequency Oscillatory Ventilation in Children: a single center experience of 53 cases. Crit Care 9:R274-R279

37. Randolph AG (2009) Management of acute lung injury and acute respiratory distress syndrome in children. Crit Care Med 37:2448-2454

38. Diaz JV, Brower R, Calfee CS, Matthay MA (2010) Therapeutic strategies for severe acute lung injury. Crit Care Med 38:1644-1650

39. Henry E, Fessler MD, Derdak S et al (2007) A protocol for high-frequency oscillatory ventilation in adults: Results from a roundtable discussion Crit Care Med Vol 35, No 7

Noninvasive Respiratory Support in Pediatrics

Cesare Gregoretti, Maria Adele Figini, Fabrizio Racca
and Edoardo Calderini

4.1 Introduction

The conventional management of acute respiratory failure (ARF) consists of endotracheal intubation; this carries potential risks, including ventilator-associated pneumonia and laryngeal-tracheal damage [1,2]. Noninvasive respiratory support (NRS) is an alternative form of respiratory treatment which incorporates various techniques aimed at improving alveolar ventilation, oxygenation, and unloading of the respiratory muscles without the need for an invasive tracheal device. Because of its safety and effectiveness, the use of NRS has been adopted throughout the world. During the last 25 years, NRS techniques have increasingly been used in the treatment of both chronic respiratory failure and ARF in adult patients in several pathological conditions. NRS applied to adults in the acute setting has been found to improve outcome, reduce the rate of intubation, and decrease the rate of complications [3].

NRS includes noninvasive continuous positive airway pressure (NCPAP) and noninvasive positive pressure ventilation (NPPV) delivered through an interface (nasal/facial mask or helmet) and high-pressure freeflow gas and turbine or piston-driven ventilators [4]. Despite the lack of a full clinical picture, in recent years NRS has been increasingly used in pediatric intensive care units and emergency departments mainly because several uncontrolled clinical trials showed improved outcomes in selected patients with ARF when compared to standard treatment. At present, NRS in children with ARF is mainly performed by experienced centers, and no universally accepted guidelines have been proposed even outside the critical care area in less severe forms of respiratory insufficiency [2]. In a review published in 2001, the authors concluded that NRS may have limited benefits in a group of carefully selected pediatric patients with acute hypoxemic and hypercarbic forms of respiratory failure [5]. However, during the last few years, its use has increased and data supporting the use of this new technique in children are growing [6–10].

C. Gregoretti (✉)
Department of Anesthesiology and Intensive Care
Azienda Ospedaliera CTO-CRF-Maria Adelaide, Turin, Italy
e-mail: c.gregoretti@gmail.com

M. Astuto (ed.) *Pediatric Anesthesia, Intensive Care and Pain: Standardization in Clinical Practice*. Anesthesia, Intensive Care and Pain in Neonates and Children
DOI: 10.1007/978-88-470-2685-8_4, © Springer-Verlag Italia 2013

4.1.1   Rationale for Noninvasive Respiratory Support

NRS, as mentioned previously, is the delivery of ventilatory support without the need for an invasive airway intervention procedure, such as endotracheal intubation or tracheotomy. The application of NRS to a patient can be "curative", as an alternative to endotracheal intubation once ARF occurs, or even "prophylactic", to prevent respiratory distress in patients who are at a higher risk of developing ARF (e.g., in postoperative and postextubation settings) or whenever the development of muscle weakness or fatigue is impending. Two types of NRS are most commonly used, i.e., NCPAP and NPPV.

The application of NCPAP takes place mainly through a high-pressure gas flow circuit, which comprises a gas circuit, a blender, a flow meter, and a positive end-expiratory pressure (PEEP) valve. Alternatively, a demand valve ventilator can be used and PEEP can be generated by high gas flows directed through a tube with increased resistance (the Coanda effect). NCPAP delivers a constant distending airway pressure throughout the entire respiratory cycle, while the patient is spontaneously breathing. It exerts its effects by: (1) increasing oxygenation and CO_2 washout by expanding collapsed alveoli and recruiting lung volume; (2) reducing the work of breathing; and (3) preventing apnea by stabilizing the upper airways and chest wall, particularly in ex pre-term babies. NPPV is extensively delivered by piston-driven or turbine ventilators. During NPPV, patients can be completely controlled by the ventilator (total controlled ventilatory support) or the patient's spontaneous inspiratory effort triggers (assisted ventilatory support) the ventilator to provide a variable volume (volume-targeted ventilation) or pressure (pressure-targeted ventilation).

During pressure-targeted ventilation the patient receives a pressure-supported flow-cycled breath (pressure support ventilation) or a time-cycled breath (assisted pressure-controlled ventilation). Unlike NCPAP, NPPV theoretically allows improved respiratory muscle unloading, alveolar recruitment, oxygenation, and CO_2 washout improvement, but patient-ventilator asynchrony may become a major issue, leading to NPPV treatment failure. Two recent physiological papers [11–12] demonstrated the effectiveness of NPPV in reducing inspiratory effort as evaluated by esophageal and transdiaphragmatic pressure-time product and esophageal tidal swings in children with ARF. In addition, the application of NPPV via nasal and/or facial mask was associated with significant improvement in breathing pattern and gas exchange.

4.1.2   Hypoxemic Acute Respiratory Failure

Hypoxemic respiratory failure is characterized by hypoxemia associated with low or normal levels of partial pressure of carbon dioxide ($PaCO_2$) in the blood. The underlying predominant mechanism is uneven or mismatched ventilation-perfusion in regional lung units. Hypoxemic respiratory failure mainly occurs in disorders characterized by parenchymal pathologies, such as bacterial and viral pneumonia, as well as in lower airway obstruction, such as bronchiolitis and status asthmaticus.

Streptococcus pneumoniae is the most common agent responsible for pneumonia, although other microorganisms can play an important role. Pneumonia produces a reduction in lung volume, due to consolidation and/or atelectasis, leading to reduced lung compliance. Bronchiolitis occurs mainly in children of less than 2 years of age and respiratory syncytial virus is estimated to be the most frequent etiological cause. Bronchiolitis causes an increase in airway resistance with dynamic lung hyperinflation, but this pathology often also involves the lung interstitium, with reduced lung volume and atelectasis. Both pneumonia and bronchiolitis can lead to acute respiratory distress syndrome (ARDS).

4.1.3 Hypercapnic Acute Respiratory Failure

The ability to breathe spontaneously is the result of a balance between neurological mechanisms controlling ventilation (central respiratory drive), together with ventilatory muscle pump power, on the one hand, and the respiratory load (resistive and elastic load), determined by the airway, lung, and thoracic elastance, on the other hand. In healthy children, the central respiratory drive and the ventilatory muscle pump exceed the respiratory load thus maintaining adequate spontaneous ventilation. However, if the force generated by the respiratory muscles pump (fatigue or weakness), or central respiratory drive is too low and/or the respiratory load is too high, the resulting alveolar ventilation may be inadequate, thus leading to hypercapnia [13]. This phenomenon can be "acute", when the imbalance is caused by an acute condition (e.g., acute exacerbation of an asthmatic patient), or "chronic", when the surge is slow during the course of a disease (e.g., a neuromuscular disease) [14,15].

4.1.4 When Should Noninvasive Respiratory Support be Used?

In adult patients, as mentioned previously, NRS has been proposed in two different contexts: (1) as a preventive or "prophylactic" application in postoperative patients to prevent ARF and extubation failure in patients at risk; and (2) as a "curative" application, once ARF occurs, to improve respiratory function and avoid endotracheal intubation. Unlike adults, to our knowledge no papers have been published to date in the pediatric literature on the use of NRS in the postoperative period. As a curative application, NRS should be initiated according to: (1) clinical signs: moderate-to-severe dyspnea and/or tachypnea (defined as a respiratory rate > the 75th percentile depending on the age of the patient); and (2) gas exchange derangement: hypoxemia [defined as a fraction of inspired oxygen (FiO_2) > 0.5 to obtain a saturation of peripheral oxygen (SpO_2) > 94%] and/or respiratory acidosis (defined as pH < 7.35). Possible contraindications for NRS are: life-threatening hypoxemia; upper airway obstruction; vomiting; cough or impaired gag reflex; facial surgery, facial trauma, or facial deformity; Glasgow Coma Scale < 10; hemodynamic instability requiring inotropes or vasopressors, or cardiac arrhythmia; and cyanotic congenital heart disease. NRS should not be started in more severe ARF in the presence of: (1) clinical signs of exhaustion (active contraction of the accessory muscles of respiration with paradoxical abdominal and thoracic motion); and (2) a PaO_2:FiO_2 ratio < 150 mmHg and/or $PaCO_2$ > 55 mmHg; and (3) pH < 7.30.

4.1.5 Noninvasive Respiratory Support in Clinical Settings

There are no data describing how to initiate NRS in children. The current knowledge is mainly based on the direct experience of clinicians working in the field, and a variety of routines are applied. Pressure target mode is by far the most common ventilatory modality in pediatric intensive care units (PICUs) [16].

However, when applying NRS via a nasal route (i.e., nasal prongs), the high nasal resistance must be taken into account. In NCPAP, PEEP pressures between 4 and 8 cm H_2O are safe and not associated with adverse hemodynamic effects. Of note, when NCPAP is delivered by helmet, a high flow system should be used to prevent CO_2 rebreathing (minimum flow rate: 30 L/min) [17]. A ventilator should never be connected to a helmet in CPAP mode.

4.1.6 Ventilators

Administering noninvasive therapeutic positive pressure ventilation is achievable through high-pressure gas flow and piston-driven or turbine ventilators. When the patient spontaneously initiates ventilation in pressure target modes, the machine is triggered and the inspiratory effort is immediately followed by the administration of a support pressure by the ventilator to reach a preset inspiratory pressure. This assumes perfect patient-machine interaction and minimal air leakage between the patient's airway and the interfaces to minimize the delay between the patient's efforts and the activation of the trigger to avoid asynchronies. Ineffective triggering and auto-triggering has been shown to be the leading cause of NRS failure due to discomfort, hyperventilation, and dynamic hyperinflation in adults [18].

The ventilator then cycles to the expiratory phase when the inspiratory flow decreases to a preset value (usually 25% of the peak inspiratory flow), as observed in pressure support ventilation, or when the patient reaches a preset inspiratory time, as observed in assisted pressure-controlled ventilation. However, during pressure support ventilation, the presence of any leak may cause the ventilator to fail to cycle to expiration causing a prolonged inspiratory time ("inspiratory hung-up"). This may cause expiratory effort, hyperinflation, discomfort, and fatigue, leading to adverse respiratory or hemodynamic consequences and NRS failure [19]. The importance of safe, comfortable, and well-fitting interfaces is mandatory to achieve success in NRS not only in pediatric patients.

In adults, ineffective inspiratory effort and double-triggering are the most common types of asynchrony leading to patient discomfort [18], whereas in children auto-triggering has been recently shown to be the primary cause of difficult patient-ventilator interaction [20].

Ueno and colleagues [21] investigated how different ventilators cope with different interface leaks. They tested three "home use" ventilators (Respironics BiPAP Vision, Respironics Trilogy 100, Murrysville, PA, USA, and Carina, Draeger, Lubeck, Germany), and two intensive care unit (ICU) ventilators (Puritan Bennett 840 Ventilator System, Covidien, Mansfield, MA, USA, and Evita XL, Draeger, Lubeck, Germany) at various positive pressure settings and leak sizes, finding that home ventilators performed better at compensating for small and medium-sized leaks. In a single-center observational prospective study, Muñoz-Bonet and colleagues [22] investigated how an ICU ventilator (Evita 2 Dura, Draeger, Lubeck, Germany) equipped with leak compensation software coped with air leaks in different modes of ventilation of pediatric patients with ARF. The study showed the effectiveness of the software in different subsets of infants and children in reducing patient-machine asynchrony. In several studies, the augmentation of trigger sensitivity, clinical observation, and the presetting of limited inspiratory time are efficient measures addressed at preventing asynchrony [8].

4.2 Interfaces

In the clinical setting, several different interfaces can be used to deliver NRS: nasal prongs, nasal masks, oronasal masks, and full-face masks. Recently, the use of a helmet has emerged and has reached immediate popularity, proving to be an effective and comfortable means of delivering positive airway pressure noninvasively [8,23], avoiding skin breakdown and other mask adverse effects [24]. Nasal prongs are typically used for the youngest patients: when directly inserted in the patient's nostrils, they are more effective for obligate nose breathers, such as newborns and young infants up to 1 year of life, in delivering continuous positive airway pressure. Normally this interface is easily kept in place without any other device, but nasal prongs are poorly tolerated for longer periods, are highly flow resistive (due to nasal anatomical resistance, to small airway resistance, and the high propensity of these patients to have hypertrophic adenoids and tonsils), and are easily obstructed by an excess of nasal secretions. Quite common side effects are bleeding, skin lesions, and nasal dryness due to airflow and nostril obstruction [3,16].

A good alternative for patients of the same age is a nasal mask. It is a small, soft and transparent mask which completely covers the nasal surface, and through which it is possible to achieve proper fitting, minimal dead space, and minimal leaks; it is therefore useful for delivering both NCPAP and NPPV. Skin lesions and mucosal breakdown are the more frequent side effects. Limitations in the use of a nasal mask include larger pressure drops due to the mouth opening [3] and the impracticability of nasogastric tube positioning [25]. In older patients (the so-called nonobligate nose breathers), oronasal masks covering both nose and mouth are more effective in minimizing air leaks and thus preserving the necessary pressurization of the respiratory system. The need for tightened straps to keep the mask in place is the main cause for patient discomfort and skin irritation. The recent introduction in the market of a full-face mask covering the entire facial surface is very promising, although no studies have been published in the pediatric population. Nasal masks, oronasal, and full-face masks need to be well-fitted to deal with leaks and discomfort, important problems that are not overcome by the use of hydrocolloid protection and that are exacerbated by facial deformities, facial trauma, and pre-existing facial lesions [8]. The recently introduced helmet is also promising in pediatric clinical practice. While its use is well established in the adult population [26,27] a few studies assessed its feasibility and effectiveness in pediatrics, both in PICUs and clinical wards, especially in acute bronchiolitis [23,28,29]. The helmet is a soft, transparent, pressurized plastic chamber that encloses the head and neck. It is easily applied in both nose and mouth breathers and in a wide range of ages and anatomical variations. Moreover, it warrants good patient-environment interaction, comfort, and reduced need for sedation in the treatment of ARF. Furthermore, the helmet allows good clearance of secretions, allows the patient to speak and swallow, and it is well tolerated for prolonged periods of application.

4.3 Predictive Factors of Noninvasive Respiratory Support Failure

NRS constitutes an alternative treatment for early pediatric ARF provided that tracheal intubation is not delayed when considered necessary. One of the major challenges during NRS is to identify the early prognostic signs of treatment failure. In a 4-year study, Muñoz-Bonet and colleagues [5] investigated several predictive factors of NRS failure in children from 1 month to 16 years of age with moderate-to-severe ARF. NRS failure was defined as the need for tracheal intubation. NRS was applied in 47 consecutive patients and failed in 9 (19.1%) due to the progression of ARF. Younger age, diagnosis of ARDS, and chest X-ray worsening at 24 h from the beginning of NRS correlated with treatment failure. The authors could also show that the association between mean airway pressure >11.5 cm H_2O and $FiO_2 > 0.6$ was predictive of NRS failure in nearly 80% of children.

In a prospective observational study, Lum and colleagues [30] investigated the factors that predict outcome of NRS in critically ill children admitted to a multidisciplinary PICU of a university hospital in Kuala Lumpur, Malaysia. Out of 278 children (average age: 8.7 months) with ARF and treated with NRS, 129 received NRS as the sole ventilatory support, 98 were treated with NRS to prevent extubation failure and 48 because of postextubation ARF. Interestingly, 71.2% of children had an underlying chronic disease, probably reflecting the typical PICU population of a developing country. Overall, NRS avoided intubation in more than 75% of children. During this study, a high pediatric risk of mortality (PRISM II) score, the presence of sepsis, an abnormal respiratory rate, and a high requirement of FiO_2 at NRS initiation were found to be independent predictive factors of NRS failure. Worsening respiratory failure and septic shock were the two leading causes of failure of NRS. The authors concluded that NRS represents an effective strategy to prevent tracheal intubation and for rapid discharge to the ward where respiratory treatment can be continued.

A high PRISM II score, a high respiratory rate, the need for oxygen, and the presence of sepsis at initiation of NRS should suggest closer monitoring to prevent NRS failure. At the Great Ormond Street Hospital in London, 163 patients aged between 1 month and 18 years who received NRS during the 7-year study period, were evaluated to determine whether physiological parameters and an underlying condition predict NRS success [31]. Eighty-three children received NRS as first-line intervention to avoid intubation and 64% of them succeeded. Those who failed showed higher FiO_2 (0.56 vs. 0.47, $p = 0.038$), higher respiratory rate (53.3 vs. 43.3 breaths/min, $p = 0.012$), and lower pH (7.26 vs. 7.34, $p = 0.032$) before NRS was started and higher FiO2 requirements once NRS was applied. Eighty patients were started on NRS to prevent postextubation failure and 60% were treated success-fully. Those individuals who failed showed significantly higher systolic and dias-tolic blood pressure 2 h after NRS start (104 vs. 77.9 mmHg, $p = 0.001$ and 64.5 vs. 54.1 mmHg, $p = 0.037$), probably representing a stress response in the wors-ening child.

Interestingly, patients on CPAP were more likely to avoid intubation when com-pared with those on bilevel positive airway pressure in both groups (first-line elec-tive and postextubation NRS). Looking at the underlying conditions, the authors demonstrated that children with a primary respiratory disease who were treated with NRS as the first-line treatment avoided intubation in 30/36 cases (83%), while those with an underlying oncological disease showed a much lower success rate (8/23 cases, 35%). The presence of sepsis further decreased the rate of success in the oncological group (3/15 cases, 20%). Patients with a primary respiratory illness were also more likely to avoid reintubation after extubation (27/33 cases, 82%). The authors concluded that tachypnea and acidosis prior to establishing NRS treatment and oxygen requirement pre- and post-NRS are the strongest predic-tive factors for treatment failure when NRS is used as the first-line treatment to prevent intubation. In contrast, when NRS is used to avoid reintubation, the most important predictive factor for reintubation is persistent hypercapnia after NRS initiation.

4.4   Conclusions

The use of NRS in the pediatric population has become an option in the last few years, and has been increasingly applied. In general, the evidence supporting its use in infants and children with ARF is still limited and the identification of the right patient, the right time of application, and the appropriate setting is still lacking, as well as universally accepted guidelines. However, the most recent physiological and randomized studies indicate that the early application of NRS can ameliorate the breathing pattern and gas exchange, and reduces respiratory muscle loading. The effects of NRS on more complex outcomes require further investigation.

To date, CPAP delivered noninvasively via a nasal mask or helmet could be considered as a first-line respiratory treatment in infants and children with mild-to-moderate ARF. NPPV applied via a facial mask probably represents the technique of choice in moderate-to-severe acute respiratory disorders, but the patient-machine interaction may become a relevant problem, particularly in younger infants. Furthermore, it is important to rely on well-trained medical and nursing staff at all times, and to apply NRS only in an ICU setting which also has appropriate cardiorespiratory monitoring.

The type of equipment and the specific ventilator settings that should be chosen remain a matter of debate. The specific equipment available for therapy evolves more rapidly with industry capability rather than with clear indications available from scientific trials.

Further studies are urgently needed to determine the criteria to initiate NPPV according to the disease profile and the age of the patient.

References

1. Orlowski JP, Ellis NG, Amin NP et al (1980) "Complications of airway intrusion in 100 consecutive cases in a pediatric ICU". Critical Care Medicine 8:324-331
2. Craven DE, Kunches LM Kilinsky V (1986) "Risk factors for pneumonia and fatality in patients receiving continuous mechanical ventilation". American Journal of Review of Respiratory Disease 133:792-796
3. Nava S, Navalesi P, Carlucci A (2009) Non-invasive ventilation. Minerva Anestesiologica 75:31-36
4. Chidini G, Gregoretti C, Pelosi P, Calderini E (2010) "Non-invasive respiratory support in children". eBook edition of Treatment Strategies-Paediatrics Cambridge Research Centre. Available online at: http://viewer.zmags.com/publication/18ab08e6"http://viewer.zmags.com/publication/18ab08e6"http://viewer.zmags.com/publication/18ab08e6
5. Muñoz-Bonet JI, Flor-Macián EM, Roselló PM et al (2010) "Predictive factors for the outcome of noninvasive ventilation in pediatric acute respiratory failure". Pediatric Critical Care Medicine 11:675-680
6. Lum LC, Abdel-Latif ME, De Bruyne JA et al (2011) "Noninvasive ventilation in a tertiary pediatric intensive care unit in a middle-income country". Pediatric Critical Care Medicine 12:e7-e13
7. Lazner MR, Basu AP, Klonin H (2012) "Non-invasive ventilation for severe bronchiolitis: analysis and evidence". Pediatric Pulmonology. Published online in Wiley Online Library (wileyonlinelibrary.com) DOI 10.1002/ppul.22513
8. Chidini G, Calderini E, Pelosi P (2010) "Treatment of acute hypoxemic respiratory failure with continuous positive airway pressure delivered by a new pediatric helmet in comparison with a standard full face mask: a prospective pilot study". Pediatric Critical Care Medicine 11:502-508
9. Essouri S, Durand P, Chevret L et al (2008) "Physiological effects of noninvasive positive ventilation during acute moderate hypercapnic respiratory insufficiency in children". Intensive Care Medicine 34:2248-2255
10. Dohna-Schwake C, Stehling F et al (2011) "Non-invasive ventilation on a pediatric intensive care unit: Feasibility, efficacy, and predictors of success." Pediatric Pulmonology 46(11):1114-1120

11. Essouri S, Durand P, Chevret L et al (2011) "Optimal level of nasal continuous positive airway pressure in severe viral bronchiolitis". Intensive Care Medicine 37:2002-2007
12. Stucki P, Perez MH, Scalfaro P et al (2009) "Feasibility of non-invasive pressure support ventilation in infants with respiratory failure after extubation: a pilot study". Intensive Care Medicine 35:1623-1627
13. Hertzog JH, Costarino AT Jr (1996) "Nasal mask positive pressure ventilation in paediatric patients with type II respiratory failure". Paediatric Anaesthesiology 6:219-224
14. Piastra M, Antonelli M, Caresta E et al (2006) "Noninvasive ventilation in childhood acute neuromuscular respiratory failure: a pilot study". Respiration 496:791-798
15. Niranjan V, Bach JR (1998) "Noninvasive management of pediatric neuromuscular ventilatory failure". Critical Care Medicine 26:2061-2065
16. Calderini E, Chidini G, Pelosi P et al (2010) "What are current indications for non invasive ventilation in children?". Current Opinion in Anaesthesiology 23(3):368-374
17. Patroniti N, Foti G, Manfio A et al (2003) "Head Helmet versus Face Mask for Non Invasive CPAP: a physiological study". Intensive Care Medicine 29:1680-1687
18. Thille AW, Rodriguez P, Cabello B et al (2006) "Patient-ventilator asynchrony during assisted mechanical ventilation". Intensive Care Medicine 32(10):1515-1522
19. Calderini E (1999) "New insights in mechanical ventilation for pediatric patients". Intensive Care Medicine 25(10):1194-1196
20. Fauroux B, Leroux K, Desmarais G et al (2008) "Performance of ventilators for noninvasive positive-pressure ventilation in children". European Respiratory Journal 31(6):1300-1307
21. Ueno Y, Nakanishi N, Oto J et al (2011) "Effects of leakage on ventilator performance during noninvasive positive pressure ventilation: a bench study". Respiratory Care 56:1758-1764
22. Muñoz-Bonet JI, Flor-Macián EM, Roselló PM et al (2010) "Noninvasive ventilation in pediatric acute respiratory failure by means of a conventional volumetric ventilator". World Journal of Pediatrics 6:323-330
23. Chidini G, Calderini E, Cesana BM et al (2010) Noninvasive Continuous Positive Airway Pressure in Acute Respiratory Failure. Helmet versus Facial Mask. Pediatrics 128:e330-e338
24. Fauroux B, Lavis JF et al (2005) "Facial side effects during noninvasive positive pressure ventilation in children." Intensive Care Medicine 31(7):965-969
25. Nørregaard O (2002) "Non invasive ventilation in children". European Respiratory Journal 20:1332-1342
26. Isgrò S, Zanella A, Sala C et al (2005) "Continuous flow biphasic positive airway pressure by helmet in patients with acute hypoxic respiratory failure: effect on oxygenation". Intensive Care Medicine 36(10):1688-1694
27. Milan M, Zanella A, Isgrò S et al (2011) "Performance of different continuous positive airway pressure helmets equipped with safety valves during failure of fresh gas supply". Intensive Care Medicine 37(6):1031-1035
28. Javouhey E, Barats A, Richard N et al (2008) "Non-invasive ventilation as primary ventilatory support for infants with severe bronchiolitis". Intensive Care Medicine 34:1608-1614
29. Yanez LJ, Yunge M, Emilfork M et al (2008) "A prospective, randomized, controlled trial of non-invasive ventilation in pediatric acute respiratory failure". Pediatric Critical Care Medicine 9:484-489
30. Lum LC, Abdel-Latif ME, De Bruyne JA et al (2011) "Noninvasive ventilation in a tertiary pediatric intensive care unit in a middle-income country". Pediatric Critical Care Medicine 12:e7-e13
31. James CS, Hallewell CP, James DP et al (2011) "Predicting the success of non- invasive ventilation in preventing intubation and re-intubation in the paediatric intensive care unit". Intensive Care Medicine 37:1994-2001

Procedural Sedation and Analgesia in Children

5

Andrea Messeri and Marinella Astuto

5.1 Introduction

Invasive and noninvasive procedures have become an essential component of modern diagnostics and therapy in children. Often, the procedures are uncomfortable and anxiety-producing for both patients and their parents. Subsequently, in the last two decades, the management of acute pain and anxiety in children undergoing brief therapeutic and diagnostic procedures outside the operating room has developed substantially. Traditionally, these were performed by anesthesiologists. Increasingly, other specialists, such as emergency room physicians, pediatricians, and radiologists, are involved in the management of procedural sedation under elective or emergency situations.

Consequently, both anesthesiologists and nonanesthesiologists are striving to provide safe and effective sedation and analgesia to these children. The availability of noninvasive monitoring, and short-acting opioids and sedatives, has broadened the possibilities of sedation and analgesia in children in diverse settings. While most of these procedures themselves pose little risk to the child, the administration of sedation or analgesia may add substantial risk to the patient. Professional organizations such as the American Society of Anesthesiologists (ASA), the American Academy of Pediatrics (AAP), the Joint Commission on Accreditation of Healthcare Organizations, and other organizations are working continuously to make procedural sedation for children safe, economical, and tailored to the needs of the child and the diagnostic/therapeutic procedure being performed. In response to published recommendations and guidelines [1–5], many institutional systems for the provision of safe procedural sedation and analgesia for children have been developed. These system models range from the use of special teams, led by anesthesiologists, intensivists, emergency physicians, or nurses that serve the entire hospital, to reliance on individual practitioners who follow sedation guidelines in their own way.

A. Messeri (✉)
Pain Management and Palliative Treatment
Meyer Children's Hospital, Florence, Italy
e-mail: a.messeri@meyer.it

M. Astuto (ed.) *Pediatric Anesthesia, Intensive Care and Pain: Standardization in Clinical Practice.* Anesthesia, Intensive Care and Pain in Neonates and Children
DOI: 10.1007/978-88-470-2685-8_5, © Springer-Verlag Italia 2013

Therefore, it is important to review the current status of sedation and analgesia for invasive and noninvasive procedures in children, providing an evidence-based approach to several topics of importance, including safety factors, patient assessment, personnel requirements, equipment, monitoring, and drugs.

5.2   Initial Considerations

When planning sedation and/or pain management for a child, knowing what level of responsiveness needs to be achieved during the procedure or test is essential for choosing the appropriate medication regimen. Painful procedures that require relative immobility generally mandate a deeper level of sedation than noninvasive radiological tests. Each sedation plan should take into account the age, developmental level, and personality of the child. A 7-year-old child, for example, may require deep sedation for the incision and drainage of an abscess; local analgesia alone may be sufficient for another child of the same age undergoing such a procedure.

One of the most important aspects of pediatric sedation and analgesia is to optimize patient safety by minimizing complications. Adverse events during sedation in children can occur owing to a variety of reasons, such as drug overdose, inadequate monitoring, drug errors, inadequate skills of the personnel administering the drugs, and premature discharge [6]. In total, 80% of the complications during sedation and analgesia are secondary to adverse airway/respiratory events [7,8]. The majority of these complications can be managed with simple maneuvers, such as providing supplemental oxygen, opening the airway, suctioning, and using bag-mask-valve ventilation. Occasionally, more advanced airway management, such as endotracheal intubation or the use of a laryngeal mask airway, is required for ventilatory assistance.

5.3   The Concept of the Continuum of the Sedation Spectrum

In an effort to clarify sedation goals, ASA defined a continuum for the levels of sedation. Minimally sedated children may have an impaired level of cognitive functioning but maintain their airway-protective reflexes and cardiorespiratory status [9,10]. For example, for children undergoing voiding cystourethrograms (VCUGs), this level of sedation is often achieved through the use of inhaled nitrous oxide. Moderate sedation is associated with blunted-but-purposeful responses to verbal or tactile stimulation. There may be subtle alterations in ventilation, but airway reflexes and cardiovascular function are generally unchanged. Infants who receive chloral hydrate often reach a moderate level of sedation. In contrast, deeply sedated children may have inadequate spontaneous ventilatory drive and/or significant upper airway obstruction and may require airway intervention. During deep sedation (as opposed to general anesthesia), purposeful responses to painful stimulation remain intact. The combination of an opioid and a benzodiazepine often results in deep sedation.

These original guidelines defined three levels of depth of sedation: conscious sedation, deep sedation, and general anesthesia. Conscious sedation was defined as a minimally depressed level of consciousness that retains the patient's ability to maintain a patent airway independently and continuously, and respond appropriately to physical stimulation and/or verbal command, for example, "open your eyes." The choice of this terminology led to confusion, as conscious sedation is rarely attained in children. In 1992, the AAP Committee on Drugs revised the 1985 guidelines [11]. They stated that regardless of the intended level of sedation or route of administration, a patient could progress from one level of sedation to another and that the provider must have the skills and equipment necessary to safely manage patients who have progressed to a deeper level of sedation. Pulse oximetry was recommended for all patients undergoing sedation.

This new guideline also discouraged the practice of parents administering sedation at home. An amendment to this guideline was published by the AAP Committee on Drugs in 2002 [5]. It eliminated the use of the term "conscious sedation." The current guidelines use the terminology of minimal sedation, moderate sedation, deep sedation, and general anesthesia to describe the continuum of the sedation spectrum (see Table 5.1).

It is vital to remember that the patient may rapidly move from one level of sedation to another (e.g., a child can move from deep sedation to either moderate sedation or to a state of general anesthesia) and, hence, personnel should have the training, in addition to the equipment, to rescue the child from deeper levels of sedation at all times when procedural sedation is provided. There are some questions raised about the concept of the sedation continuum, as it relies on subjectivity in identifying and quantifying a patient's response to verbal or tactile stimulation. This subjectivity may vary among observers and it is not logical to apply this to patients who may be unable to respond appropriately, for example, patients with hearing impairments, developmental delay, neurological compromise, or at extremes of age. In the future, it may be possible to reformulate the sedation continuum by shifting away from subjective assessment to more objective vital signs monitoring, through focused research and the development of a multidisciplinary sedation community to help define the stages of sedation.

Table 5.1 The continuum of the sedation spectrum

	Minimal sedation axiolysis	Moderate sedation (conscious sedation)	Deep sedation	General anesthesia
Response	Responds normally to verbal commands	Responds purposefully to verbal commands or light touch	Responds to pain	No response
Airway	Maintained	Maintained	May require support	May be necessary
Cardiovascular support	Not needed	Not needed	May be needed	May be necessary

Perhaps the most important factor for ensuring safety during pediatric procedural sedation is the immediate availability of skilled rescue resources. Adverse pediatric sedation events are most common in facilities that lack adequately trained personnel and reliable emergency response support. Physicians should carefully consider the following questions before embarking on a sedation plan:

1. What is the skill set of the team that will be with the child at all times?
2. If the primary team needs help, who will respond?
3. How long will it take the rescue team to arrive?
4. Is a member of the rescue team an anesthesia specialist who is capable of providing reliable advanced airway support to children?
   Satisfactory answers to these questions are critical to ensuring safety.

Following the implementation of the 2001 Joint Commission on Accreditation of Healthcare Organizations guidelines, the incidence of adverse events during procedural sedation has been markedly reduced [12]. Adherence to AAP/ASA guidelines for pediatric procedural sedation may reduce the adverse events, and there is direct evidence that elements of the AAP/ASA structural model for procedural sedation could be adopted by nonanesthesiologists with an apparent risk reduction [13].

5.4   Patient Evaluation

What "red flags" should providers look for when evaluating a child who would benefit from sedation for a painful or anxiety-provoking procedure? Although identifying every possible risk factor can be challenging even for the most seasoned pediatric anesthesiologist, there are specific patient characteristics that have been associated with increased complications. A thorough health history and physical examination can reveal many of them.

First, the provider should find out why the child is having the procedure or test. The provider should then find out whether the child has medical issues that could put them at increased risk for complications. Recent upper respiratory illness symptoms, especially coughing, wheezing, or nasal congestion, can increase the risk of airway irritability and respiratory complications, including hypoventilation, desaturation, and laryngospasm. Similarly, a history of recent vomiting or symptomatic gastroesophageal reflux can be cause for concern, as emesis during sedation, when airway-protective reflexes may be blunted, could lead to aspiration and initiate laryngospasm. Significant obesity, an increasing problem in the pediatric population, may be associated with an increased risk of airway obstruction, especially with deeper levels of sedation. Overt obstructive sleep apnea symptoms are clearly associated with airway obstruction during sedation; however, many families are unable to say how frequently or how badly their children snore. Even occasional audible snoring makes the need for airway repositioning and nasopharyngeal airway placement more likely.

Physicians should also be aware of underlying medical conditions that increase the potential for airway compromise during sedation. A number of genetic syndromes are associated with anatomic and/or developmental airway differences as well as altered respiratory mechanics; several excellent articles describe these [14,15]. Infants born prematurely have immature respiratory drive physiology, increasing the likelihood of sedation-related apnea in the first months of life. Currently, many sedation programs choose to monitor infants less than 60 weeks postconceptual age for a longer time period than they do older children prior to discharge. For example, at Children's Hospitals and Clinics of Minnesota, we monitor these infants for a 12-h period, discharging them to home only if they have not had any episodes of apnea during that time. Changes in respiratory physiology during procedural sedation can aggravate underlying asthma or bronchopulmonary dysplasia, potentially leading to bronchospasm and/or desaturation.

Physical examination should focus on findings that could affect the course of the child's sedation. The physician should look for craniofacial abnormalities that could be problematic if the patient should need bag-mask ventilation or endotracheal intubation. These include, but are not limited to, facial anomalies such as retrognathia that can prevent good mask seal and interfere with airway visualization, tonsillar hypertrophy that can prevent adequate air entry, and limited neck mobility that can prevent adequate airway positioning. Physicians should also remember to look for braces and other orthodontia. Many neuromuscular disorders are associated with decreased ability to handle oral secretions; these secretions can pool in the hypopharynx and lead to coughing, laryngospasm, or aspiration when airway reflexes are blunted. Children who have obvious wheezing or other respiratory difficulties should have their test or procedure rescheduled. If the procedure or test is deemed to be an emergency, an anesthesia consultation should be sought. Significant abdominal distension can increase the risk of vomiting and aspiration.

Although the need for strict nothing by mouth (NPO) guidelines for urgent and emergent sedations continues to be a topic of debate, most physicians should plan to adhere to the recommended ASA guidelines [1]. These suggest the following NPO times:
- Clear liquids: 2 h
- Breast milk: 4 h
- Infant formula, other nonhuman milk, solids: 6 h
- Full meal: 8 h

For children requiring sedation who do not meet the ASA NPO guidelines, recommended options include delaying the procedure or seeking an anesthesia consultation [16]. The literature suggests that the aspiration risk for procedural sedation and analgesia is lower than that of general anesthesia because the principal risk factors (airway manipulation, absence of protective airway reflexes, and poor ASA physical status) are not present routinely in this setting [17,18]. As a reflection of this evidence, some emergency physicians disregard preprocedural fasting guidelines. However, even though published studies suggest that strict adherence to the fasting guidelines is not necessary, their sample size and/or designs are insufficient to safely practice the liberalized preprocedural fasting guidelines and to justify changes in emergency department procedural sedation and analgesia policies.

5.5 Preparation and Setup for Sedation and Analgesia

The single best way to monitor a sedated child is continuous direct observation by one or more trained providers not directly involved with the procedure itself. Beyond this basic tenet, the frequency and intensity of monitoring depend on the depth of the sedation being performed. At a minimum, all sedated patients should be monitored with continuous pulse oximetry. The ASA also recommends that respiratory function be continuously monitored by observation, auscultation, and/or capnography. Electrocardiography (ECG) should be used and blood pressure (BP) should be measured intermittently during deep sedation.

Equipment needs are based on patient management and rescue. A number of mnemonics can help the sedation provider remember the essentials; one of the most popular is the SOAPME mnemonic:
- suction: appropriately sized large-bore suction catheters, smaller catheters for nasal or endotracheal suctioning, functional vacuum apparatus;
- oxygen: adequate supply, functioning flow meters;
- airway equipment: appropriately sized masks, self-inflating or anesthesia bag-valve-mask (BVM) systems, nasopharyngeal and oropharyngeal airways, laryngeal mask airways, laryngoscope blades and handles, endotracheal tubes;
- pharmacy: sedative analgesic medications, reversal agents, emergency resuscitation, and airway medications;
- monitors: pulse oximetry, cardiorespiratory monitor with ECG and BP capability, stethoscope, end-tidal carbon dioxide monitor; and
- extras: intravenous access catheters, isotonic resuscitation fluid, emergency drug sheet, calculator.

The type of procedure being performed may also dictate other equipment needs. Documentation of sedation encounters should include informed consent, postsedation instructions, and contact information for the parent or guardian. A focused history and physical examination should be performed and documented at the time of sedation. The plan for procedural sedation as well as an assessment of the child's sedation risks and ASA classification should be included in the documentation. A time-based recording of vital signs, sedation scores, and administered medications is required. Also, any adverse events and associated interventions should be noted.

5.6 Personnel and Training

The provider responsible for sedation in pediatric patients must be familiar with monitoring, as per the AAP guidelines, and competent in managing the complications. The sedation may exceed the intended level and the provider should be sufficiently skilled to rescue the child from a deeper level of sedation. The provider must be trained in and capable of providing BVM ventilation and advanced airway skills if required, to keep the child oxygenated. At least one individual must be present who is trained in advanced pediatric life support. Human simulators offer an extremely promising technology in the promotion of the safe administration of pediatric procedural sedation. This technology will train the sedation providers to recognize the critical airway emergencies and initiate resuscitation. The study [19] carried out to measure the system safety and errors supports the feasibility of using available human simulation.

5.7   Vascular Access and Monitoring

Children receiving deep sedation should have an intravenous access placed at the start of the procedure. An intraosseous needle should be available in the event of failure to place an intravenous line, or if the intravenous line becomes nonfunctional in an emergency situation. If the child is receiving sedative agents other than via the intravenous route, for example, intranasal, oral, or rectal, the need for intravenous access is debatable. Most authors recommend the placement of intravenous access for the administration of emergency medications, including reversal agents, during procedural sedation.

Prior to administration of sedative medication, a baseline determination of vital signs should be documented. The selection of medication with appropriate concentration and labeling is essential to prevent medication errors [7]. Medications with minimal effect on respiration are associated with fewer respiratory adverse events [20], and titration of the medication dose guided by the bispectral index (BIS) may be useful in preventing oversedation [21]. Continuous monitoring of oxygen saturation, heart rate, and respiratory rate using capnography and intermittent measurement of BP should be documented. The new-generation pulse oximeters are less susceptible to motion artifacts. Oximeters that change the tone with changes in hemoglobin saturation provide immediate aural warning to everyone within hearing distance. The oximeter probe must be properly positioned; clip-on devices can be easily displaced and could result in a false reading. Capnography is valuable in monitoring respiration, especially in children sedated in less accessible locations, such as during a magnetic resonance imaging (MRI) or computerized tomography (CT) scan, or in darkened rooms. Nasal cannulae that allow the simultaneous delivery of oxygen and measurement of expired CO_2 are very useful in making the diagnosis of airway obstruction or apnea during sedation. In a recent randomized controlled trial, investigators examined the use of a capnography monitor during emergency department sedation using propofol and opioids in adults [22]. They concluded that the addition of capnography to standard monitoring reduces hypoxic events and also provides early warning of the development of hypoxemia. Capnography has been demonstrated to improve patient safety during procedural sedation by reducing the apnea/hypoxia events [23]. Any restraining devices should be checked to prevent airway obstruction or restriction of chest movement.

5.8 Sedatives and Analgesics: a Difficult Choice

A number of medications are used for pediatric procedural sedation. There is rarely a right or wrong choice with regard to medication selection; however, the physician's familiarity and experience with various agents are important considerations. Many of the more commonly used sedation agents have no analgesic component, so adding a medication for pain control or choosing a different regimen may be more appropriate for painful procedures.

Benzodiazepines have been a mainstay of procedural sedation for many years. A drug in this class can be used as a single agent for brief, nonpainful procedures and as an adjunct in combination with opioids or ketamine for more painful ones. The pharmacokinetics of midazolam make it most suited for procedural sedation. Onset of action occurs in less than 60 s when administered intravenously (IV), and its duration is usually a few minutes. Midazolam may be administered via many different routes: IV, orally, rectally, or intranasally. Although the combination of midazolam and an opioid analgesic can provide excellent sedation and analgesia for painful procedures, the combination is also associated with a higher incidence of respiratory depression.

Nitrous oxide, a longtime favorite sedative/analgesic agent for dental procedures, is becoming increasingly popular as a minimally sedating agent for a variety of pediatric procedures, including IV catheter placements, VCUGs, lumbar punctures, and other brief, painful procedures. Nitrous oxide is delivered as either a fixed 50/50 mixture with oxygen or in titratable concentrations of 30–70%. Onset of action generally takes place within 2–3 min, and its effect rapidly ends when the gas is discontinued. Nitrous oxide may also be combined with an opioid analgesic for more painful procedures such as joint taps, but this combination can induce moderate or even deep levels of sedation. The incidence of nausea and vomiting following nitrous oxide administration is approximately 5% [9]. Challenges with inhalation equipment and appropriate waste anesthetic gas scavenging have limited the use of nitrous oxide in some locations.

Chloral hydrate has been used as a sedative hypnotic agent for more than 100 years. It is particularly useful for inducing a sleep state in children younger than 2 years of age for a nonpainful procedure such as a CT/MRI scan or an auditory brain stem response (ABR) test for hearing. Chloral hydrate is administered orally, with an onset of action usually within 20–30 min, although onset of action can be somewhat variable. Duration of action can be even more unpredictable. Most children sleep for 60–120 min, but the long elimination half-life of chloral hydrate occasionally can result in prolonged sedation states that can last more than 12 h. Because of the unpredictable duration of action, there have been reports of serious adverse events and even death following discharge for children who received chloral hydrate for sedation [10]. Rates for successful sedations are between 85% and 95%. In rare instances, younger children never achieve the depth of sedation required to complete the associated procedure. The rate of failed sedation increases markedly for children over the age of 3 years. Although chloral hydrate administration is generally associated with a moderate level of sedation and rarely with respiratory depression, the incidence of respiratory complications is higher in infants, especially those younger than 2 months of age [24].

Barbiturates, most commonly pentobarbital, have also been mainstays of sedation for nonpainful pediatric procedures in the past. Although the use of pentobarbital has been largely supplanted by newer agents such as propofol and dexmedetomidine, it is still used for moderate sedation for procedures such as MRI scans. The advantages of pentobarbital include its 1–2 min IV onset time, the ability to provide repeat dosing in as little as 5–10 min, and limited respiratory and hemodynamic effects in otherwise healthy children. However, children with underlying respiratory or cardiovascular issues may be more susceptible to associated cardiopulmonary instability. Although children can become quite deeply sedated, and even anesthetized, with pentobarbital, it does not provide any analgesic effects. The disadvantages of using pentobarbital for procedural sedation include its potential for prolonged deep sedation and unpredictable recovery time, which can range from 60 min to more than 12 h, as well as its association with recovery dysphoria and agitation (unaffectionately labeled "pentobarb rage") [25].

Dexmedetomidine is a relatively new, highly selective central alpha-2 adrenergic receptor agonist with both sedative and analgesic properties. Already in use as an intensive care unit sedative analgesic, dexmedetomidine has migrated to the procedural sedation arena, where it is a preferred agent for many providers because of its limited effects on respiration. Dexmedetomidine is generally associated with a moderate level of sedation that, according to electroencephalogram (EEG), mimics normal sleep. Therefore, many pediatric neurologists prefer dexmedetomidine for children who require sedation for successful completion of EEGs. Dexmedetomidine has also proven to be useful for the sedation of children with autism or other developmental concerns, as the recovery period seems to be associated with a much less troublesome emergence [26]. Most often, dexmedetomidine is administered as an IV agent, with a slow initial bolus over 5–10 min followed by a continuous infusion; it also can be given orally or buccally with good success. Dexmedetomidine can be associated with clinically significant cardiovascular effects, especially bradycardia, because of its effects on cardiac conduction times.

Many children's hospitals have built their sedation programs around the sedative/anesthetic agent propofol. By far the most commonly used agent for pediatric procedural sedation, it is used both as a single agent for nonpainful procedures such as CT, MRI, and ABR testing, and in combination with analgesics such as ketamine and fentanyl for a variety of painful procedures. Propofol is administered intravenously and its many advantages include onset in 30–60 s, offset generally in 5–15 minutes, and ease of titration to effect. For longer procedures, bolus propofol is used for induction, and deep sedation is maintained by a continuous IV infusion. Propofol use is associated with a high incidence of respiratory depression and induction can easily lead to rapid loss of airway reflexes and apnea [27]. Physicians who administer propofol must be able to rescue patients from a general anesthetic state and have expertise in both BVM ventilation and endotracheal intubation. Because of the risk of rapid respiratory decompensation, some hospitals restrict the use of propofol to anesthesia providers. In addition, propofol can lead to bradycardia and hypotension, although these effects are typically mild and do not become clinically significant in otherwise healthy children.

For decades, opioids have been the most commonly administered analgesic medications. Although they have no inherent amnestic qualities and limited sedative effects when used independently, they may be used in combination with sedative/hypnotic agents to facilitate deep sedation for painful procedures. Fentanyl is the most commonly used procedural opioid because of its pharmacokinetic profile and low cost. The onset of an IV dose of fentanyl occurs within 2–3 min, with peak effect at 5 min. This more rapid onset allows for more titratable dosing for procedural analgesia than morphine, which has an onset of action of 5–10 min. As with all opioids, fentanyl leads to dose-dependent respiratory depression, especially when used in combination with another sedative agent.

Ketamine is a favorite medication to facilitate sedation for painful procedures in the emergency department. Ketamine is a derivative of phencyclidine and it is uniquely associated with sedative, dissociative, amnestic, and analgesic properties. At lower doses, ketamine leads primarily to anxiolytic and analgesic effects. With higher doses, ketamine produces antegrade amnesia and a dissociative state of sedation/anesthesia. On awakening, children often report having experienced very vivid dreams or hallucinations. Ketamine may be administered via IV, intramural, oral, rectal, or nasal routes. Deep levels of sedation are generally achieved. Typically, patients maintain spontaneous respiratory drive and adequate airway-protective reflexes, although ketamine is a sialagogue, and the additional saliva it produces can increase the risk for laryngospasm. Ketamine also leads to increased heart rate, BP, and cardiac output in previously hemodynamically stable children. Unique side effects associated with ketamine include a potential increase in intracranial and intraocular pressure as well as negative neuropsychiatric effects with emergence delirium and significant agitation. The incidence of vomiting with ketamine sedation ranges from 12% to 25% but does seem to be decreased with the coadministration of midazolam and/or ondansetron.

5.9   Postsedation Recovery and Discharge

Ongoing monitoring and observation are critical during recovery from procedural sedation and should continue until the child's vital signs and level of interaction have returned to their presedation baselines. Significant adverse events can occur during emergence, especially if medications with longer half-lives were used. The recovery area should be equipped with the same monitoring and resuscitation equipment as the sedation and procedural area itself, and the same rescue resources should be available. Children should be discharged only when they have met specific pre-established recovery criteria and after the family has received detailed instructions for postsedation care, including instructions on how to seek follow-up medical care if needed.

5.10 Conclusions

Pediatric sedation requires careful consideration of the balance between the patient's risk factors, the procedure being performed, and the provider's experience and expertise. With appropriate preparation, physicians can offer safe and effective procedural sedation to meet the needs of their pediatric patients.

Sedation and analgesia in children for procedures outside the operating room are rapidly expanding, and are being driven to be more cost-effective and efficient. Highly motivated and organized sedation/anesthesia services are likely to reduce serious adverse outcomes, but minor adverse events are actually common. The majority of the adverse events associated with pediatric sedation and analgesia are respiratory/airway-related, which can be managed with simple maneuvers. There should be a real collaboration between the anesthesiology department and other concerned departments to enhance the safe and effective management of pediatric sedation and analgesia outside the operating room.

5.11 Future Developments

With the increasing frequency of diagnostic and therapeutic procedures in children, the demand for sedation and analgesia for children outside the operating room setting is exceeding the capacity of anesthesia services. The number of children requiring sedation outside the operating room may approach the number of children requiring anesthesia in the operating room in 5 years time, and as a result, more nonanesthesiologists could be asked to provide procedural sedation outside the operating room. Hospitals are likely to set up multidisciplinary pediatric sedation teams that will not only administer procedural sedation, but will also be responsible for training and credentialing for all nonanesthesiologists in procedural sedation. The anesthesiology department should collaborate with other providers and establish structured training involving human simulation, with emphasis on critical events. There is a need for pharmacological agents with minimal respiratory and cardiovascular depression; newer drugs such as the alpha-2 adrenergic receptor agonist dexmedetomidine offer significant advantages and huge potential for widespread use. The use of brain function monitors, such as the BIS, and respiratory monitors, such as end-tidal CO_2 monitoring, will be routinely used to provide safe and effective sedation. Results from the pediatric sedation research consortium and other studies could help us identify strategies to prevent and manage adverse events during procedural sedation in children.

References

1. Krauss B (2000) Sedation and analgesia for procedures in children. N Engl J Med 342(13): 938-945
2. Krauss B, Green SM (2006) Procedural sedation and analgesia in children. Lancet 367(9512): 766-780
3. Joint Commission on Accreditation of Health Care Organizations (2000) Comprehensive Accreditation Manual for Hospitals. JCAHO, Oakland, IL, USA
4. American Society of Anesthesiologists. Task Force on Sedation and Analgesia by Non-Anes-thesiologists (2002) Practice guidelines for sedation and analgesia by non-anesthesiologists. Anesthesiology 96(4):1004-1017
5. American Academy of Pediatrics. Committee on Drugs (2002) Guidelines for monitoring and management of pediatric patients during and after sedation for diagnostic and thera-peutic procedures: addendum. Pediatrics 110(4):836-838
6. Malviya S, Voepel-Lewis T, Tait AR (1997) Adverse events and risk factors associated with the sedation of children by nonanesthesiologists. Anesth. Analg 85(6):1207-1213
7. Cote CJ, Karl HW, Notterman DA et al (2000) Adverse sedation events in pediatrics: analy-sis of medications used for sedation. Pediatrics 106(4):633-644
8. Cote CJ, Notterman DA, Karl HW (2000) Adverse sedation events in pediatrics: a critical incident analysis of contributing factors. Pediatrics 105(4 Pt 1):805-814
9. Guidelines for the elective use of conscious sedation, deep sedation, and general anesthesia in pediatric patients. Committee on Drugs (1985) Section on anesthesiology. Pediatrics 76(2):317-321
10. Goodson JM, Moore PA (1983) Life-threatening reactions after pedodontic sedation: an as-sessment of narcotic, local anesthetic, and antiemetic drug interaction. J Am Dent Assoc 107(2):239-245
11. American Academy of Pediatrics Committee on Drugs (1992) Guidelines for monitoring and management of pediatric patients during and after sedation for diagnostic and therapeutic procedures. Pediatrics 89(6 Pt 1):1110-1115
12. Pitetti R, Davis PJ, Redlinger R et al (2006) Effect on hospital-wide sedation practices af-ter implementation of the 2001 JCAHO procedural sedation and analgesia guidelines. Arch Pediatr Adolesc Med 160(2):211-216
13. Hoffman GM, Nowakowski R, Troshynski TJ (2002) Risk reduction in pediatric procedur-al sedation by application of an American Academy of Pediatrics/American Society of Anes-thesiologists process model. Pediatrics 109(2):236-243
14. Butler MG, Hayes BG, Hathaway MM et al (2000) Specific genetic diseases at risk for se-dation/anesthesia complications. Anesth Analg 91(4):837-855
15. Butler MG, Hayes BG, Hathaway MM et al (2001) Congenital malformations: the usual and the unusual. ASA Refresher Courses in Anesthesiology 29:123-133
16. Green SM (2003) Fasting is a consideration – not a necessity – for emergency department procedural sedation and analgesia. Ann Emerg Med 42(5):647-650
17. Green SM, Krauss B (2002) Pulmonary aspiration risk during emergency department pro-cedural sedation – an examination of the role of fasting and sedation depth. Acad Emerg Med 9(1):35-42
18. Roback MG, Bajaj L, Wathen JE, Bothner J (2004) Preprocedural fasting and adverse events in procedural sedation and analgesia in a pediatric emergency department: are they related? Ann Emerg Med 44(5):454-459
19. Blike GT, Christoffersen K, Cravero JP (2005) A method for measuring system safety and latent errors associated with pediatric procedural sedation. Anesth Analg 101(1):48-58, table of contents
20. Roback MG, Wathen JE, Bajaj L, Bothner JP (2005) Adverse events associated with pro-cedural sedation and analgesia in a pediatric emergency department: a comparison of com-mon parenteral drugs. Acad Emerg Med 12(6):508-513

21. Powers KS, Nazarian EB, Tapyrik SA et al (2005) Bispectral index as a guide for titration of propofol during procedural sedation among children. Pediatrics 115(6):1666-1674
22. Deitch K, Miner J, Chudnofsky CR (2010) Does end tidal CO_2 monitoring during emergency department procedural sedation and analgesia with propofol decrease the incidence of hypoxic events? A randomized, controlled trial. Ann Emerg Med 55(3):258-264
23. Qadeer MA, Vargo JJ, Dumot JA et al (2009) Capnographic monitoring of respiratory activity improves safety of sedation for endoscopic cholangiopancreatography and ultrasonography. Gastroenterologies 136(5):1568-1576; quiz 1819-1820
24. Litman RS, Soin K, Salam A (2010) Chloral hydrate sedation in term and preterm infants: an analysis of efficacy and complications. Anesth Analg 110(3):739-746
25. Mallory MD, Baxter AL, Kost SI et al (2009) Propofol vs pentobarbital for sedation of children undergoing magnetic resonance imaging: results from the Pediatric Sedation Research Consortium. Pediatr Anesth 19(6):610-611
26. Lubisch N, Roskos R, Berkenbosch JW (2009) Dexmedetomidine for procedural sedation in children with autism and other behavior disorders. Pediatr Neurol 41(2):88-94
27. Cravero JP, Beach ML, Blike GT et al (2009) The incidence and nature of adverse events during pediatric sedation/anesthesia with propofol for procedures outside the operating room: a report from the Pediatric Sedation Research Consortium. Anesth Analg 108(3):795-804

The "Open" Intensive Care Unit: the Challenge Continues

6

Alberto Giannini

Restricting visiting in ICUs is neither caring, compassionate, nor necessary.
Donald M. Berwick and Meera Kotagal, JAMA (2004)

6.1 Introduction

Nearly 10 years have passed since Hilmar Burchardi, past president of the European Society of Intensive Care Medicine, wrote in an editorial in *Intensive Care Medicine* that "it is time to acknowledge that the ICU must be a place where humanity has a high priority. It is time to open those ICUs which are still closed [1]".

The intervening period of time has undeniably brought about some changes in the direction indicated by Burchardi, but the "opening" of intensive care units (ICUs) even if no longer a "dream" is certainly still far from being a full "reality".

The literature gives a patchy picture of visiting policies in the critical care setting. The latest available percentages of adult ICUs without restrictions on visiting hours are 70% in Sweden [2], 32% in the USA [3], 23% in France [4], 22% in the UK [5], 14% in Netherlands [6], and 3.3% in Belgium [7]. Italian ICUs overall maintain very restrictive visiting policies. However, over the last 5 years, in Italy there has been perceptible change in this field: daily visiting time has essentially doubled (from 1 to around 2 h) and there has been a substantial increase in ICUs allowing 24-h visiting (from 0.4% to 2%) [8,9].

As regards children, well into the 1960s their admission into hospital inevitably entailed their separation from parents and family [10,11]. Visiting was severely restricted or even prohibited, being considered dangerous or simply of no value. Aspects such as disruption of the intrinsic bond between child and parents or the loss of the parental role were practically unknown or disregarded as irrelevant. As for pediatric ICUs (PICUs), a US study in 1994 showed that 57% of 125 units restricted visits to brief daily periods [12]. Another North American study found that eight PICUs out of 12 limited visits to varying extents and that only two had an unrestricted visiting policy [13]. In Italian PICUs, the median daily visiting time

A. Giannini (✉)
Pediatric Intensive Care Unit, Fondazione IRCCS Ca' Granda – Ospedale Maggiore Policlinico, Milan, Italy
e-mail: a.giannini@policlinico.mi.it

M. Astuto (ed.) *Pediatric Anesthesia, Intensive Care and Pain: Standardization in Clinical Practice*. Anesthesia, Intensive Care and Pain in Neonates and Children
DOI: 10.1007/978-88-470-2685-8_6, © Springer-Verlag Italia 2013

for parents is currently 5 h; 12% of units have unrestricted policies and 59% do not allow the constant presence of a parent even during the day [14].

6.2   The Liberalization of Visiting Policies in Intensive Care Units

6.2.1   The Case in Favor

For many doctors and nurses the term "open" ICU still represents a kind of oxymoron, i.e., literally an unreal condition in which noun and adjective are in clear and irreconcilable opposition. This point of view is largely consistent with past history. From the time of their creation less than 50 years ago and for many years thereafter, ICUs were "closed" wards where access for family members and visitors was looked on unfavorably and was therefore strictly limited. This strategy was frequently motivated above all by fears regarding the risk of infection, interference with patient care, increased stress for patients and family members, and the violation of confidentiality [1,15].

So, for many years admission of a patient to ICU followed what we might call a "revolving door principle", i.e., when the patient came in, their family was sent out. The logic behind this entrenched behavior was that the strategic objective of prime importance, i.e., the life and health of the patient, justified resorting to a kind of "sequestration" of that patient. The reduction or abolition of contacts with the patient's affective world was considered a reasonable price to pay to obtain the far greater advantage of life and health themselves.

However, not only are the reasons for restricting visits groundless [1,15], but there are strong arguments in favor of liberalizing access to the ICU for patients' families. Current knowledge has shown that separation from loved ones is a significant cause of suffering for the ICU patient [16,17], and that for the family to be allowed to visit at any time represents one of the most important needs [18–20]. On this subject, it is interesting to note that ICU doctors and nurses largely underestimate [17,21] both the need of the sick person to have their loved ones nearby and the relatives' need for information and proximity (which are the main needs of families of ICU patients, together with assurance, support, and comfort) [19–21].

Regarding the pediatric world specifically, separation from their parents has long been recognized as the greatest source of stress for hospitalized young children [22]. From the point of view of the parents, in addition to uncertainty regarding their child's condition and outcome, a major source of stress is the loss of their parental role [22]. Being with the child is, together with frequent and accurate information about their condition, the most important need of parents; often their priority is not constant presence at the child's bedside but the freedom to visit their child when they can or wish to [23].

Separation from loved ones is often for the patient a further and unjustified "price to pay" on top of the illness or acute event which caused the admission to ICU.

Alongside the patient's suffering there is also that of their family, which is often not recognized or given scant consideration: for example, symptoms of anxiety and depression were found in 73% and 35% of family members, respectively [24]. Moreover, post-traumatic stress symptoms consistent with a moderate-to-major risk of post-traumatic stress disorder (PTSD) were found in 33% of family members [25]. It is important to stress that the suffering of families is not a transitory event but can in fact persist long after the patient is discharged. Evidence of this is that at 6–12 months after discharge, 27% of parents of PICU-admitted children were assessed to be at high risk for PTSD (as compared with 7% of parents of ward-admitted children) [26].

Numerous data suggest that the liberalization of access to ICU for family members and visitors [18,27] is not only in no way dangerous for patients, but is on the contrary beneficial both for them and for their families. In particular, an unrestricted visiting policy causes no increase in septic complications [28,29], while cardiocirculatory complications, anxiety scores, and hormonal stress indicators are significantly lower [28]. It also has the positive effect of sharply reducing anxiety in the families of patients [30]. For instance, mothers of children admitted to an "open" PICU have lower stress indicators than those of children in a PICU with "limited access" [31].

6.2.2 Visiting by Children

Children visiting family members who have been taken into intensive care, is also, under certain conditions, a positive and welcome occurrence. On this subject, a nationwide multicenter study in Sweden found that all the ICUs covered by the study had a positive policy regarding visits by children to adult patients, though 34% of the wards had some *de facto* restrictions in place [2]. Moreover, it should be considered that there are no real reasons for systematically discouraging visits by siblings to children admitted into intensive care: the presence of a sister or brother has a positive and reassuring effect on the patient. Apart from certain specific exceptions (e.g., when the visitor has a contagious infection), if the child is suitably prepared and supported by the family context (and by other "powerful" contexts, such as their school), the visit to an ill sibling helps to dispel the children's fears and fantasies of loss or death, and reassures them of their parents' continuing attention [11].

6.2.3 Procedures and Cardiopulmonary Resuscitation

A recent survey found that in Italian PICUs there is a clear tendency to substantially limit the presence of parents during procedures (even ordinary nursing ones) and cardiopulmonary resuscitation [14]. In 38% of units parents were not normally allowed to be present at the bedside during ordinary nursing procedures such as endotracheal suctioning. In the case of invasive procedures such as inserting a central venous catheter and in the case of cardiopulmonary resuscitation, the presence of parents was permitted only in 3% and 9% of units, respectively.

This topic has recently been reviewed by Dingeman and colleagues [32]: most parents wish to have the option to remain with their child during invasive procedures and resuscitation, and those who have done so would repeat their choice in the future. Parents can calm or emotionally support their child and help caregivers. Moreover, reduced anxiety and help with the grieving process are two of the main benefits for parents permitted to be present during procedures or resuscitation.

Although the presence of family members during resuscitation has been recommended [33], it is not unanimously considered a positive thing and continues to raise concerns among physicians and nurses [34,35].

6.3 The "Open" Intensive Care Unit

6.3.1 Ethical Aspects

There is in fact no solid scientific basis for limiting visitors' access to ICUs [1,15,18,27]. Moreover, on both ethical and clinical grounds, only serious public health risks can exceptionally justify restricting visits [36].

Even in the area of health, the choices we make, the reasons behind them, and the actions that result must be weighed up to assess their acceptability on an ethical level. The philosopher Emmanuel Levinas wrote [37] that the capacity to recognize "the face of the other" generates responsibility towards, and relationship with, them. It is possible and it is fitting to transpose these terms – responsibility and relationship – even into the complex environment of intensive medicine, giving rise to new gestures and language. It is in this perspective that the choice of the "open" ICU makes sense also on an intrinsically ethical level and thus it becomes necessary, precisely because it more fully addresses not only the needs of the other, but also the valuing of, and respect for, that person's life.

Another element to be considered in the area of ethical aspects – certainly for adults and teenagers – is respect for autonomy. We must clear up a misunderstanding here. In allowing the presence of family and visitors in the ICU, we doctors and nurses are not making any concession to the patient. Instead, with this action we recognize a clearly defined right of the patient. The patient – where this is feasible – should be given the option to decide which people are particularly significant for them and who they therefore wish to have nearby in the difficult period of sickness. A significant proportion of admissions to the ICU is not triggered by sudden or acute events, but rather these are scheduled events (major surgery, transplants) or represent a predictable stage in the progression of a chronic disease (oncological, cardiac, respiratory, neurological, and so on). There is therefore plenty of scope for consulting patients as to their wishes so that they may decide in advance which visitors are important to them.

6.3.2   Experience in the Field

With the knowledge that liberalization of visiting hours offers beneficial effects for both patient and family, the necessity of "opening" ICUs has been pointed out authoritatively and repeatedly [1,15,18]. In particular, it has been recommended that visiting in PICUs should be open to parents 24 h a day [18]. However, from the picture outlined previously, we may deduce that in many countries there is not yet a full awareness that the presence of loved ones at the bedside is beneficial for the patient and that in the critical care setting family is actually a resource rather than a hindrance [38,39].

The experience of units that have already liberalized their visiting polices provides some interesting information. A French study, for example, highlights three issues [40]. First, the median visit length is around 2 h a day and the majority of family visits are mostly concentrated in the afternoon and evening (so there is not a sort of "invasion" of ICU). This probably happens because relatives, despite this period of particular difficulty and suffering, still have to face – sometimes having to resort to complex juggling – all the commitments imposed by normal working and family life. Second, neither nurses nor physicians perceive open visitation as disrupting patient care (even though it may induce moderate discomfort among nurses due to possible interference with patient care). Finally, most family members report that the 24-h policy lessened their anxiety. In addition, a recent Italian survey found that most ICU staff members view the "opening" of the unit positively, and on the whole maintain this opinion 1 year after the policy change [41].

6.3.3   Not Just a Question of Time

The liberalization of visiting policies is only one aspect of a more complex issue and the author would like to propose a shift in perspective. Creating the "open" ICU is not just a question of time: we also need to consider "openness" in terms of physical and relational dimensions. The "physical dimension" includes all the barriers recommended to or imposed on the visitor, such as no physical contact with the patient, gowning procedures (of no value in infection control [1]), and so on The area of "relationships" involves the communication – often fragmentary, compressed, or even nonexistent – among ICU staff, patient, and family. If we also address these aspects, an "open" ICU may be defined as a unit in which one of the caregivers' objectives is a carefully considered reduction or elimination of any limitations imposed on these three dimensions (temporal, physical, and relational) for which there is no justified reason [42,43].

Being able to see the work carried out in the ICU with their own eyes thus helps to give the family reassurance, strengthening their conviction that their loved one is being properly looked after around the clock. In addition, "open" access makes for better communication [27] with nurses and doctors as well as increasing the family's trust in and appreciation of the care team. It may inevitably be that, in certain circumstances, family members exhibit an "overvigilant" or even hostile attitude [27], which may be in response to a closed stance adopted by the ICU team (in the form of restricting information, excluding family from the decision-making process on key issues, and so on). It is in the interests of the patient that these relationships be carefully restored to mutual trust and respect.

6.3.4 A New Language

Working in the ICU and the endeavor to create a patient-centered ICU [18,44] can be enriched with new words and actions. For instance, the terms "welcome" and "hospitality" are rich and evocative ways of referring to the way we relate to the other, even in the context of a hospital. They can be "inflected" in the specific reality of the ICU and translated into behavior or attitudes. An "open" ICU offers the possibility to devise new gestures and language, rich in humanity. A first example pertains to the "body": touching the patient's body, holding them (even if still intubated and on a ventilator, or on noninvasive ventilation), feeding the patient a little, and so on, are gestures of enormous value both on the level of the relationship and on the therapeutic level. An effort is required to create the conditions to make this possible, with all due safeguards, but it must be made evident that the patient's body is not something "expropriated" and inaccessible to loved ones.

We live in a society which does not like to "see people die," which censors death and hides it away. But no area of medicine highlights as critical care does that the practice of medicine is governed by limits. Almost every day in the ICU staff touch the limit with their hand and must look death in the face. In the light of the considerations explored previously as to what an "open" ICU means and the reasoning behind it, "death" too may be approached in a different way, with a different "language" and gestures from the customary ones. We are generally accustomed to the gesture of "delivering a body" after death, but we can instead create the conditions whereby "the person is accompanied" at the time of death. The semantic and symbolic difference is obvious, but experience shows that there is also a profound practical difference between the two. Providing the circumstances permit it and if death is not an acute and unexpected event, it is important to allow relatives to be with their loved one even in the terminal phase of life, staying close by, touching, caressing (or holding them, in the case of a child), speaking to them with their own intimate gestures and words. These are heartrending, unutterable moments – literally "unspeakable" – but of enormous importance. Moreover, all these gestures of leave-taking represent the first step on the way to working through the grieving process.

6.3.5 Tackling the Difficulties

"Open" ICUs may therefore provide fuller and more appropriate responses to some of the needs of patients and their families. However, it would be wrong to play down the difficulties or inconveniences involved in an innovative choice such as this. These are for the most part associated with habits and "cultural" aspects, which constrain both the medical team and the patient's family. We should also bear in mind that personality traits or habits such as obtrusiveness, aggressiveness, or mistrust almost always tend to be exacerbated by new, stressful situations such as the serious illness of a family member. This whole matter is often dealt with in a rigid fashion, with reference more to the regulations (a true "totem" of hospital life) than to the meaning of the events and a search for balanced and rational solutions.

An "open" ICU does not, however, mean an ICU "without rules" [42], and it is both practical and necessary to draw up some guidelines. Visitors should be required not only to show the greatest consideration for all the patients in the unit, but also to follow some basic rules concerning hygiene (e.g., to wash their hands before and after the visit); security (e.g., not to touch equipment or vascular access lines); and operations (e.g., to move out of the way during emergency maneuvers). Each individual ICU may draw up its own rules and modify them over time on the basis of a critical assessment of their own operations. It is also important to give the medical team time and space of their own, allowing free communication and full respect of confidentiality, but also some indispensable breaks not constantly punctured by interruptions.

Finally, we should not deny or underestimate the possible difficulties that ICU staff face (particularly nurses) in opening the unit, mainly to do with a different style of relations with visitors and the burden for staff members of learning to work under the eyes of family members.

6.3.6 The Way Forward

In the author's view, there are at least four courses which we must now pursue [43]. The first concerns information and education of ICU physicians and nurses. We must invest time and resources in increasing knowledge of and sensitization to these issues (visiting policies, patient and family needs, patient-centered ICUs, and so on) among caregivers.

Second, there is also a great need for research into these issues and, in particular, investigation of any difficulties which liberalizing visiting could cause for ICU staff (e.g., anxiety, stress, and overwork). It is essential to create a picture of the problems and understand their causes and extent, to identify possible solutions and offer nurses and physicians appropriate support.

Third, communication skills must be fully recognized as a specific area of professional competency for ICU caregivers, which needs to be improved or updated. In addition, as recently recommended [18], ICU staff should also receive training in conflict management, meeting facilitation skills, and assessment of family needs and family members' stress and anxiety levels. Today, the cultural baggage of the intensivist can no longer be limited exclusively to practical "know-how": in the care of the ICU patient, clinical skills and familiarity with technology are a necessary but not sufficient condition. Finally, unrestricted visiting should be made a requirement for a hospital's accreditation in the public health service.

6.4   Conclusions

Despite the many objections considered valid until recently (mainly infection risks, interference with patient care, increased stress for patient and family members, violation of confidentiality), there is no sound scientific basis for limiting visitors' access to critical care units. There is now wide consensus that the liberalization of visiting in ICUs/PICUs is a useful and effective strategy to respond to the needs of patients and their families. However, the "open" ICU is not just a question of visiting time: we also need to consider "openness" in terms of physical and relational dimensions.

It is not always easy to "open" our ICUs. It necessarily involves disrupting the rhythms and rules of a well-established and reassuring tradition. It is a choice which commits us to coming up with original solutions for each individual situation, which will require regular monitoring, and need to be renewed and remotivated over time. But what is needed above all is a certain degree of cultural change and serious consideration regarding the value and quality of relationships with patients and their families.

References

1.   Burchardi H (2002) Let's open the door! Intensive Care Med 28:1371-1372
2.   Knutsson SE, Otterberg CL, Bergbom IL (2004) Visits of children to patients being cared for in adult ICUs: policies, guidelines and recommendations. Intensive Crit Care Nurs 20:264-74
3.   Lee MD, Friedenberg AS, Mukpo DH et al (2007) Visiting hours policies in New England intensive care units: strategies for improvement. Crit Care Med 35:497-501
4.   Lautrette A, Darmon M, Megarbane B et al (2007) A communication strategy and brochure for relatives of patients dying in the ICU. N Engl J Med 356:469-478
5.   Hunter JD, Goddard C, Rothwell M et al (2010) A survey of intensive care unit visiting policies in the United Kingdom. Anaesthesia 65:1101-1105
6.   Spreen AE, Schuurmans MJ (2011) Visiting policies in the adult intensive care units: a complete survey of Dutch ICUs. Intensive Crit Care Nurs 27:27-30
7.   Vandijck DM, Labeau SO, Geerinckx CE et al (2010) An evaluation of family-centered care services and organization of visiting policies in Belgian intensive care units: a multicenter survey. Heart Lung 39:137-146
8.   Giannini A, Miccinesi G, Leoncino S (2008) Visiting policies in Italian intensive care units: a nationwide survey. Intensive Care Medicine 34:1256-1262
9.   Giannini A, Marchesi T, Miccinesi G (2011) "Andante moderato": signs of change in visiting policies for Italian ICUs. Intensive Care Medicine 37:1890
10. Giganti AW (1998) Families in pediatric critical care: the best option. Pediatr Nurs 24:261-265
11. Page NE, Boeing NM (1994) Visitation in the pediatric intensive care unit: controversy and compromise. AACN Clin Issues Crit Care Nurs 5:289-295
12. Whitis G (1994) Visiting hospitalized patients. J Adv Nurs 19:85-88
13. Tughan L (1992) Visiting in the PICU: a study of the perceptions of patients, parents, and staff members. Crit Care Nurs Q 15:57-68
14. Giannini A, Miccinesi G (2011) Parental presence and visiting policies in Italian pediatric ICUs: a national survey. Pediatric Critical Care Medicine 12:e46-e50

15. Berwick DM, Kotagal M (2004) Restricted visiting hours in ICUs: time to change. JAMA 292:736-737
16. Nelson JE, Meier DE, Oei EJ et al (2001) Self-reported symptom experience of critically ill cancer patients receiving intensive care. Crit Care Med 29:277-282
17. Biancofiore G, Bindi ML, Romanelli AM et al (2005) Stress-inducing factors in ICUs: what liver transplant recipients experience and what caregivers perceive. Liver Transpl 11:967-972
18. Davidson JE, Powers K, Hedayat KM et al (2007) Clinical practice guidelines for support of the family in the patient-centered intensive care unit: American College of Critical Care Medicine Task Force 2004-2005. Crit Care Med 35:605-622
19. Molter NC (1979) Needs of relatives of critically ill patients: a descriptive study. Heart Lung 8:332-339
20. Leske JS (1986) Needs of relatives of critically ill patients: a follow-up. Heart Lung 15:189-193
21. Bijttebier P, Vanoost S, Delva D et al (2001) Needs of relatives of critical care patients: perceptions of relatives, physicians and nurses. Intensive Care Med 27:160-165
22. Melnyk BM (2000) Intervention studies involving parents of hospitalized young children: an analysis of the past and future recommendations. J Pediatr Nurs 15:4-13
23. Kasper JW, Nyamathi AM (1988) Parents of children in the pediatric intensive care unit: what are their needs? Heart Lung 17:574-581
24. Pochard F, Darmon M, Fassier T et al (2005) Symptoms of anxiety and depression in family members of intensive care unit patients before discharge or death. A prospective multicenter study. J Crit Care 20:90-96
25. Azoulay E, Pochard F, Kentish-Barnes N et al (2005) Risk of post-traumatic stress symptoms in family members of intensive care unit patients. Am J Respir Crit Care Med 171:987-994
26. Rees G, Gledhill J, Garralda ME et al (2004) Psychiatric outcome following paediatric intensive care unit (PICU) admission: a cohort study. Intensive Care Med 30:1607-1614
27. Slota M, Shearn D, Potersnak K et al (2003) Perspectives on family-centered, flexible visitation in the intensive care unit setting. Crit Care Med 31(5 Suppl):S362-S366
28. Fumagalli S, Boncinelli L, Lo Nostro A et al (2006) Reduced cardiocirculatory complications with unrestrictive visiting policy in an intensive care unit: results from a pilot, randomized trial. Circulation 113:946-952
29. Malacarne P, Corini M, Petri D (2011) Health care-associated infections and visiting policy in an intensive care unit. Am J Infect Control 39:898-900
30. Simon SK, Phillips K, Badalamenti S et al (1997) Current practices regarding visitation policies in critical care units. Am J Crit Care 6:210-217
31. Proctor DL. (1987) Relationship between visitation policy in a pediatric intensive care unit and parental anxiety Child Health Care 16:13-17
32. Dingeman RS, Mitchell EA, Meyer EC et al (2007) Parent presence during complex invasive procedures and cardiopulmonary resuscitation: a systematic review of the literature. Pediatrics 120:842-854
33. Fulbrook P, Latour J, Albarran J et al (2008) The presence of family members during cardiopulmonary resuscitation. Paediatr Nurs 20:34-36
34. O'Brien MM, Creamer KM, Hill EE et al (2002) Tolerance of family presence during pediatric cardiopulmonary resuscitation: a snapshot of military and civilian pediatricians, nurses, and residents. Pediatr Emerg Care 18:409-413
35. Waseem M, Ryan M (2003) Parental presence during invasive procedures in children: what is the physician's perspective? South Med J 96:884-887
36. Rogers S (2004) Why can't I visit? The ethics of visitation restrictions – lessons learned from SARS. Crit Care 8:300-302
37. Lévinas E (1985) Ethics and infinity. Duquesne University Press, Pittsburgh
38. McAdam JL, Arai S, Puntillo KA (2008) Unrecognized contributions of families in the intensive care unit. Intensive Care Med 34:1097-101

39. Garrouste-Orgeas M, Willems V, Timsit JF et al (2010) Opinions of families, staff, and patients about family participation in care in intensive care units. J Crit Care. 25:634-640
40. Garrouste-Orgeas M, Philippart F, Timsit JF et al (2008) Perceptions of a 24-hour visiting policy in the intensive care unit. Crit Care Med 36:30-35
41. Giannini A, Miccinesi G, Prandi E et al (2012) 'Opening' ICU: views of ICU doctors and nurses before and after liberalization of visiting policies. Critical Care 16(Suppl 1):P492
42. Giannini A (2007) Open intensive care units: the case in favour. Minerva Anestesiol 73:299-305
43. Giannini A (2010) The "open" ICU: not just a question of time. Minerva Anestesiol 76:89-90
44. Carlet J, Garrouste-Orgeas M, Dumay MF et al (2010) Managing intensive care units: Make LOVE, not war! J Crit Care 25:359.e9-359.e12

Long-Term Home Ventilation in Children: Advances and Perspectives

7

Fabrizio Racca, Cesare Gregoretti, Elena Capello, Cristina Bella, Ida Salvo, Edoardo Calderini and Marco Ranieri

7.1 Introduction

Long-term mechanical ventilation (LTMV) has been defined as the need for mechanical ventilation delivered via tracheotomy (invasive mechanical ventilation) or noninvasive interfaces (noninvasive ventilation, NIV), including continuous positive airway pressure (CPAP), for at least 3 months after its commencement, for a minimum amount of 6 h per day, in medically stable conditions [1,2]. A recent Italian study showed that all LTMV users received invasive or noninvasive positive pressure ventilation (NPPV) and only 1.5% of children were also managed with other ventilatory assistance modes (i.e., 1% with glossopharyngeal breathing and 0.5% with phrenic nerve stimulation) [1].

Over the past 20 years, LTMV in the pediatric population has rapidly expanded [1–7]. This has been attributed to a number of factors: (1) continuous advances in neonatal and pediatric intensive care are likely to result in a greater number of children with critical chronic conditions, who survive and are discharged home, but who require long-term technological support [4]; (2) a growing population of children exists who have chronic respiratory failure (CRF) due to conditions such as neuromuscular disorders (NMDs), obstructive sleep apnea, or craniofacial abnormalities; (3) LTMV for children with NMDs and chest wall disorders is an established supportive therapy that reduces morbidity and mortality [8–11]; and (4) manufacturing development (i.e., mechanical ventilators and noninvasive interfaces) has made NIV a practical option even for very young children [4].

It is now accepted practice that the home environment is preferable to the hospital setting once the decision to institute LTMV in an infant or child with a stable or progressive disorder of the respiratory system has been taken [12]. In fact, LTMV at home offers the best option for the child's psychosocial development, social

F. Racca (✉)
Pediatric Anesthesiology and Intensive Care Unit,
SS. Antonio Biagio e Cesare Arrigo Hospital, Alessandria, Italy
e-mail: fabrizio.racca@gmail.com

M. Astuto (ed.) *Pediatric Anesthesia, Intensive Care and Pain: Standardization in Clinical Practice*. Anesthesia, Intensive Care and Pain in Neonates and Children
DOI: 10.1007/978-88-470-2685-8_7, © Springer-Verlag Italia 2013

integration, and quality of life. Moreover, the direct cost of home care is usually lower than that of hospital care [12]. As matter of fact, several surveys have shown that the majority of children on LTMV are successfully discharged home [1–3,7].

The aim of this chapter is to discuss some of the issues and problems arising from home mechanical ventilation in children.

7.2   The Rationale for the Use of Long-Term Mechanical Ventilation

The ability to sustain spontaneous breathing can be viewed as a balance between neurological mechanisms controlling ventilation and respiratory muscles power on the one hand, and the respiratory load determined by lung, thoracic, and airway mechanics on the other. In healthy children, the central respiratory drive and respiratory muscle power exceed the respiratory load; thus, they are able to sustain adequate spontaneous ventilation. Significant dysfunction of any of these three components of the respiratory system may impair the ability to generate spontaneously efficacious breaths. If respiratory load is too high and/or respiratory muscle power or the central respiratory drive is too low, ventilation may be insufficient, resulting in alveolar hypoventilation and hypercapnic CRF [12].

Several factors make very young children more susceptible than adults to develop respiratory failure [12,13]. Because of pulmonary and chest wall mechanics (i.e., a relatively stiff lung and a very compliant chest wall), respiratory load is increased. The compliant chest wall also impedes the ability to generate adequate tidal volumes (TVs). The mechanics of the respiratory system are further hampered by high-flow resistance of the nasal airway and small airways. Reduced respiratory muscle strength and endurance increase a child's susceptibility to fatigue. In addition, in young children the neurological control of breathing is an intrinsically unstable system, which predisposes to apnea and hypoventilation. Finally, the formation of alveoli is essentially complete by 18 months and the metabolic rate in very young children is approximately twice that of adults, thus increasing the risk of hypoxemia. If the respiratory imbalance leading to hypercapnic CRF cannot be corrected with medical treatment, ventilator support may be indicated.

Infants and children may require LTMV due to one or more of three categories of respiratory system dysfunction: (1) increased respiratory load (due to intrinsic pulmonary disorders or skeletal deformities); (2) respiratory muscle weakness (due to neuromuscular diseases or spinal cord injury); or (3) failure of the neurological control of ventilation (central hypoventilation syndrome) [12] (see Table 7.1). The majority of children on LTMV have NMDs [1–3,6,7] and the most represented NMDs are spinal muscular atrophy [1] and congenital myopathy [7].

The decision to initiate LTMV in a pediatric patient may be undertaken electively or non-electively [12]. In the past, most decisions to begin LTMV were made *non-electively*. LTMV was started as a result of weaning failure after the institution of mechanical ventilation in the acute setting. More recently, the decision to

Table 7.1 Causes of chronic respiratory insufficiency in pediatric patients

1. Increased respiratory load	1.1 Chronic pulmonary disorders	1.1.1 Upper airway obstruction: obstructive sleep apnea; craniofacial syndromes; airway malacia; vocal cord paralysis; Prader-Willi syndrome; obesity syndromes; Down syndrome; achondroplasia 1.1.2 Chronic lung disease: bronchopulmonary dysplasia; lung hypoplasia; cystic fibrosis
	1.2 Chest wall disorders	Severe kyphoscoliosis; thoracic dystrophy; other thoracic wall deformities
2. Ventilatory muscle weakness	2.1 Neuromuscular disorders	2.1.1 Motoneuron diseases: spinal muscular atrophy (SMA); SMA with respiratory distress 2.1.2 Peripheral neuropathies: phrenic nerve paralysis; Guillain-Barré syndrome; chronic inflammatory demyelinating polyneuropathy 2.1.3 Neuromuscular junction diseases: myasthenia gravis (MG); congenital autoimmune MG; congenital myasthenias 2.1.4 Muscle diseases: *Progressive muscular dystrophies*: Duchenne muscular dystrophy; myotonic dystrophy *Congenital muscular dystrophies*: Ullrich congenital muscular dystrophy (CMD); Bethlem myopathy; Emery-Dreifuss dystrophy; merosin-deficient CMD alpha-dystroglycanopathies *Congenital myopathies*: central core disease; nemaline rod myopathies; centronuclear/myotubular myopathy; fiber-type disproportion myopathy; myofibrillar myopathies *Metabolic myopathies*: mitochondrial encephalomyopathies; glycogen storage disorders (GSDs; i.e.; GSD type II or Pompe disease); lipid storage myopathies
	2.2 Spinal cord injury (above C3):	Traumatic spinal cord injury; tumor; surgery
	2.3 Encephalopathy	Birth injury; cerebral palsy
3. Ventilation control failure	3.1 Congenital central hypoventilation:	– Congenital central hypoventilation syndrome (Ondine's curse) – Late-onset central hypoventilation syndrome – Rapid-onset obesity with hypothalamic dysfunction; hypoventilation, and autonomic dysregulation
	3.2 Acquired central hypoventilation	Trauma; tumor; surgery; hemorrhage; radiation; myelomeningocele; Arnold-Chiari type II

CMD congenital muscular dystrophy, *GSD* glycogen storage disorder, *MG* myastenia gravis, *SMA* spinal muscular atrophy

start LTMV is increasingly being made *electively* to preserve physiological function. In this case, LTMV is aimed at: (1) unloading the respiratory muscles; (2) decrease hypercapnia during wakefulness; (3) reduce fatigue and improve respiratory muscle performance; (4) preserve normal pulmonary mechanics; (5) improve nutritional status; (6) avoid chest wall distortion; (7) preserve normal growth; (8)

increase sleep quality; (9) facilitate airway clearance during physiotherapy; (10) reduce hospitalizations and intensive care unit care; and (11) improve quality of life [12,13]. Finally, in patients with NMDs and chest wall disorders, LTMV has been shown to reduce morbidity and mortality [8–11].

When the decision to initiate LTMV is taken electively, ventilatory support is usually applied first during the night. This is due to several factors: (1) an increase in upper airway resistance due to a decrease of tonic activity of the upper airway muscles occurs during rapid eye movement (REM) sleep; (2) a reduction in respiratory pump performance during REM sleep due to the reduced activity of intercostal muscles coupled with a preserved activity of the diaphragm; (3) a fall in functional residual capacity leading to an increase in ventilation-perfusion mismatch; and (4) a modification of the central drive due to an alteration of chemoreceptor sensitivity during sleep.

LTMV nocturnal beneficial effects may be extended, after prolonged use, during diurnal spontaneous breathing. These effects may be due to an increase in respiratory drive caused by a reduction in cerebrospinal fluid bicarbonate concentration which resets the ventilatory response to CO_2. Moreover, an improvement in sleep quality influences respiratory muscle endurance [14].

7.3   Criteria for Home Discharge

Once a child, who started LTMV non-electively, has become clinically stable both in terms of underlying disease symptoms and ventilator settings, they have become a candidate for LTMV given at home. Indeed, with proper patient selection, home care is safe and optimizes the patient's quality of life, rehabilitative potential, and reintegration with the family [12].

However, the child who is going to be discharged to home care should present the following conditions: (1) respiratory system stability; (2) ventilator requirement stability; (3) stability of other medical conditions for a relatively sustained period of time (1–2 weeks); and finally (4), it must be considered if the current level of care can be continued at home [12].

Respiratory system stability means that children should meet the following stability criteria:

1. The child should have safe and secure airways (i.e., either tracheostomy with a sufficient mature stoma to allow tube changes, or stabilized on regimen of NIV with minimal risk for aspiration).
2. The child should be able to clear secretions, either spontaneously or with assistance (i.e., manually or mechanically assisted coughing).
3. The child should not have episodic severe dyspnea nor sustained episodes of moderate dyspnea.
4. The child should have stable airway resistance and lung compliance.
5. Oxygenation should be stable including during suctioning and tracheostomy repositioning.

Ventilator requirement stability means that:

1. The child should have stable ventilator settings on the ventilator in use and defined type of respiratory circuits;
2. The child should have stable fraction of inspired oxygen (FiO_2) ≤ 0.4 with positive end-expiratory pressure (PEEP) ≤ 5 cm H_2O (unless on higher PEEP for obstructive sleep apnea);
3. The child, ideally, should be able to do some ventilator-free breathing.

Stability of other medical conditions means that all other medical problems should be controlled and that there are no major diagnostic considerations or changes in therapeutic interventions requiring hospitalization within 1 month (i.e., treatment plan for all medical conditions is in place, will not require frequent changes, and can be implemented at home). Furthermore, an adequate nutrition program is in place, preferably through the enteral route.

Finally, to continue at home the current level of care, the child should have: (1) stable home and family setting; (2) a home environment prepared in advance to accommodate their needs; and (3) caregivers identified and trained to provide the necessary care prior to discharge.

7.4   When to Start Elective Long-Term Mechanical Ventilation

Elective LTMV is started when spontaneous respiratory muscle efforts are unable to sustain adequate alveolar ventilation. If reversible deteriorating factors (i.e., respiratory infection, heart failure, severe electrolyte disturbance) have been treated successfully, indications for elective LTMV include symptomatic or nonsymptomatic daytime hypercapnia, symptomatic or nonsymptomatic nocturnal hypoventilation, failure to thrive, recurrent chest infections, paradoxical breathing, and chest wall deformity [8,9,15–18]. The criteria for selecting children with CRF to receive elective LTMV are listed in Table 7.2.

In children with spinal muscular atrophy (SMA) type 1, care without ventilation support is an option if the burden of treatment outweighs the benefits. If supportive ventilation is chosen by the family, NIV is recommended. In fact, for these patients, tracheotomy is controversial and an ethical dilemma. On the other hand, NIV can be used as a palliative to facilitate discharge from hospital to home and to reduce the work of breathing [8,17].

Respiratory status in patients with CRF is assessed primarily with *pulmonary function tests* [8,9,15]. Spirometry in sitting and supine positions is of particular importance as a difference greater than 20% between the sitting and supine vital capacity is indicative of diaphragmatic weakness and suggests a higher risk of nocturnal hypoventilation. Moreover, a sitting vital capacity that is lower than 40% of the predicted value is indicative of nocturnal hypoventilation [15]. An oronasal mask allows children with facial weakness to achieve a reliable value for vital capacity. For patients unable to perform standard spirometry because of young age or developmental delay, a crying vital capacity can be obtained by placing a

Table 7.2 Criteria for the selection of children with CRF for long-term mechanical ventilation

Nocturnal ventilation is indicated in patients who have any of the following:
- significant daytime CO_2 retention ($PaCO_2 > 45$–50 mmHg while awake);
- signs or symptoms of hypoventilation (patients with FVC < 30% predicted are at especially high risk);
- significant nocturnal hypoventilation ($PtcCO_2 \geq 50$ mmHg for > 10% of nocturnal recording time or $PtcCO_2 \geq 50$ mmHg for at least 5 continuous min) or significant oxygen desaturation (SpO_2 was < 90% for > 10% of nocturnal recording time or SpO_2 was $\leq$ 90% for at least 5 continuous min, or four or more episodes of SpO_2 < 92%, or drops in SpO_2 of at least 4% per h of sleep) or an apnea-hypopnea index > 10 per h on polysomnography;
- failure to thrive;
- recurrent chest infections (> 3 a year);
- paradoxical breathing and chest wall deformity (above all in children with SMA type 1).

In patients already using nocturnally assisted ventilation, daytime ventilation is indicated for:
- self-extension of nocturnal ventilation into waking hours;
- abnormal swallowing due to dyspnea, which is relieved by ventilatory assistance;
- inability to speak a full sentence without breathlessness;
- symptoms of hypoventilation with significant daytime CO_2 retention ($PaCO_2 > 45$–50 mmHg while awake).

CRF chronic respiratory failure, *FVC* forced vital capacity, *PaCO₂* partial pressure of oxygen (in the blood), *PtcCO₂* transcutaneous CO_2, *SpO₂* oxygen saturation, *SMA* spinal muscular atrophy

tightly fitting mask on the nose and mouth with a spirometer in line [15]. Maximal inspiratory pressure and maximal expiratory pressure are additional measures of pulmonary function. Values < 60 cm H_2O suggest respiratory impairment.

Arterial or capillary blood gases assess hypercapnic respiratory failure (i.e., a partial pressure of CO_2, $PaCO_2$) in the blood > 45 mmHg). Sleep studies are used to evaluate nocturnal respiratory compromise [8, 15]. In particular, polysomnograms can detect or confirm sleep-disordered breathing and should include end-tidal CO_2 monitoring or transcutaneous CO_2 monitoring. When polysomnography is not available, an alternative is to use a 4-channel sleep study that records heart rate, nasal airflow, and chest wall movements during sleep. In cases where neither polysomnography nor a 4-channel study is available, overnight pulse oximetry with continuous CO_2 monitoring may provide useful information about nighttime gas exchange [8].

Furthermore, a proactive approach should be taken to recognize the "early symptoms of pulmonary problems" prior to the onset of chronic respiratory compromise. Early symptoms can be subtle and may include disturbed sleep, increased need to turn at night, waking in the morning feeling tired, disturbed mood, irritability and poor concentration during the day, morning headaches, nausea, fear of going to sleep, and nightmares. These symptoms are typically related to nighttime hypercapnia and hypoxemia. However, the onset of hypoventilation may be insidious and patients may be clinically asymptomatic [8].

Repeated chest infections, accessory muscle use, tachypnea, presence of paradoxical breathing, swallowing difficulties, and poor weight gain or weight loss can also be signs of pulmonary impairment [8,15].

Additional screening tests should include a baseline chest X-ray to provide an initial reference point and for comparison during respiratory deterioration or unexplained hypoxemia due to unsuspected atelectasis. Moreover, formal evaluation of swallowing should be considered in patients with NMDs if clinically indicated or in cases of an acute unexplained respiratory deterioration and recurring pneumonia [8]. Finally, children with NMDs should be evaluated for the presence and severity of scoliosis [8].

7.5   How to Deliver Long-Term Mechanical Ventilation

LTMV can be delivered in the home setting as noninvasive CPAP or as intermittent positive pressure ventilation (IPPV) [12].

CPAP applies a constant distending airway pressure throughout the entire respiratory cycle, while the patient is breathing spontaneously. CPAP exerts its effects in patients with CRF by: (1) splinting the upper airway; (2) stabilizing the chest wall; (3) counterbalancing the intrinsic PEEP; (4) recruiting lung volume and maintaining inflated collapsed alveoli; and (5) reducing the cardiac afterload.

Invasive or noninvasive IPPV assists ventilation during inspiration by delivering pressurized gas to the airways, increasing transpulmonary pressure, and inflating the lungs. Exhalation occurs by means of elastic recoil of the lungs with or without active force exerted by the expiratory muscles. IPPV exerts its effects in patients with CRF by: (1) increasing alveolar ventilation; (2) unloading respiratory muscles; and (3) relieving the patient's dyspnea.

During IPPV, ventilators can deliver a positive pressure breath regardless of the patient's inspiratory drive (total ventilator-controlled mechanical support: "controlled mechanical ventilation") or in synchrony with the patient's effort (partial patient-controlled mechanical support modes: "assisted mechanical ventilation"). In the "assisted modes", the patient's spontaneous inspiratory effort triggers the ventilator to provide a volume (volume-targeted ventilatory modes) or pressure (pressure-targeted ventilatory modes).

Volume-targeted ventilation (VTV) is characterized by the delivery of a predetermined TV. The main advantage of this mode is that a minimal volume is guaranteed. On the other hand, pressure being the dependent variable, high inspiratory airway pressures may cause discomfort and poor tolerability [19]. Moreover, this mode is less efficient in compensating for air leaks than pressure-targeted ventilation.

Differently from VTV, during pressure-targeted ventilation the independent variable is pressure, while flow is the dependent variable. As a consequence, TV is not predetermined, depending on the level of pressure, patient's inspiratory effort, and the mechanical properties of the respiratory system (i.e., resistance and compliance). Pressure-targeted ventilation includes assist-control pressure-targeted ventilation and pressure support ventilation (PSV). During assist-control pressure-targeted ventilation each breath may be triggered by the patient's effort and terminated at a given time. Patients control the respiratory rate, but the breath is always time-cycled. The ventilator set-up always asks for a backup rate and for ventilator inspiratory time (usually 33% of the patient's duty cycle). During PSV each breath is triggered by the patient's effort and terminated at a given preset or adjustable threshold of the patient's inspiratory flow decay (i.e., the termination criteria). Therefore, in this mode patients can control both the respiratory rate and the inspiratory duration [20]. Even if during genuine PSV there are no mandatory breaths present, home ventilators frequently have a PSV mode incorporating a backup rate to prevent episodes of apnea.

New turbine-driven ventilators can be set on VTV or pressure-targeted ventilation, and integrate new options such as "pressure-targeted ventilation with closed-loop control", which guarantees a minimal TV. The principle of this "volume guarantee" module is based on the automatic detection of the TV by the ventilator. When the TV falls below a fixed threshold, the ventilator increases the inspiratory positive pressure or inspiratory flow and eventually the inspiratory time until the delivered TV is reached. After the resolution of a pathological condition (i.e., an increase in airway resistance), the ventilator should be able to return to its baseline settings while preserving the patient's ventilator synchrony.

The optimal mode for LTMV has not been established. Therefore, the choice between ventilatory modes is determined by the type of the underlying disease and the habits of the prescriber. However, the majority of patients with tracheostomy are managed with VTV or pressure-targeted ventilation with "volume guarantee," reflecting the common practice of using ventilation modalities with a guaranteed TV even in case of changes in resistance (i.e., secretions, tube plugging, and so on) [1]. In addition, VTV may be required for patients with advanced restrictive disease, such as NMD patients, in whom daytime mouthpiece ventilation may be necessary. Indeed, mouthpiece ventilation can only be performed with a volume-targeted mode. Finally, VTV may be preferred in patients with NMDs because of their ability to "stack" breaths to assist cough. On the other hand, children with chronic lung disease noninvasively ventilated are preferentially assisted with pressure-targeted ventilation, which may compensate for air leaks, by varying the inspiratory flow, and which enhances patient comfort resulting in higher treatment "compliance" [1]. Finally, CPAP is almost exclusively applied as a first-line therapy in patients with upper airway obstruction [1].

Once the ventilator mode is chosen, the optimal setting for LTMV has to be established. In general, mechanical ventilation settings are individualized to achieve adequate inspiratory chest wall expansion and air entry, and the normalization of oxygen saturation (SpO_2) and end-tidal CO_2 or transcutaneous CO_2 measurements. For children without significant pulmonary disease, ventilators are adjusted to provide an end-tidal CO_2 partial pressure (pCO_2) of 30–35 mmHg and $SpO_2 > 95\%$ [12]. In these patients, the partial pressure of CO_2 in the blood ($PaCO_2$) should be adjusted slightly lower than the physiological $PaCO_2$ (i.e., 30–35 mmHg) to provide a margin of safety and eliminate subjective feelings of dyspnea [12]. For children with pulmonary disease, these low pCO_2 values may not be achievable, and supplemental oxygen may be required, in addition to mechanical ventilation, to achieve adequate oxygenation [12].

The level of positive pressure required to eliminate obstructive apneas or hypopneas and normalize ventilation and nighttime SpO_2 must be determined in the sleep laboratory or with careful bedside monitoring and observation.

Patient-ventilator asynchrony may become a major issue during the "assisted modes" leading to mechanical ventilation failure. Essouri and colleagues found that CPAP and NIV were associated with a significant and comparable decrease in respiratory effort in infants with upper airway obstruction. However, NIV ventilation was associated with patient-ventilator asynchrony [21].

At home, ventilator settings cannot be changed frequently to maintain perfect blood gas values. Thus, settings should not be changed in response to minor variations in blood gas values, but only to correct persistent trends or major abnormalities.

Once the child is at home, serial evaluation and adjustment of LTMV are necessary, as the child grows and as patient's requirements change with time. Consequently, ventilator settings must be evaluated to assure adequate gas exchange (pulse oximetry, capnography, transcutaneous pO_2 and pCO_2) on a regular basis. Generally, these evaluations should be performed more frequently in infants and small children with rapid growth, and less frequently in older children with slower growth. In preschool children, ventilator settings should be checked every 4–8 months. After the fourth year of life, ventilator settings should be checked every 6–12 months [12]. Furthermore, following any change in the respiratory system (such as severe infection or hospitalization), ventilator settings should be checked and readjusted.

7.6 Characteristics of Home Ventilators

Some home ventilators are pressure-targeted, others volume-targeted, and new turbine-driven ventilators contains both modes and can be set on different modalities, such as CPAP and PSV, as well as VTV and assist pressure control ventilation (APCV), with or without PEEP. Furthermore, some home ventilators are able to deliver "intentional leak" ventilation by using a single circuit with manufactured leaks [such as CPAP or bilevel positive airway pressure (BiPAP), others can deliver "non-leak" ventilation by using a single circuit with an expiratory valve or a double circuit, and several new ventilators contain both these modalities.

"Intentional leak" ventilation is very effective in compensating for additional leaks. This ability is very important in the case of NIV. Furthermore, using NIV, the choice between leak and non-leak ventilation is also determined by the type of underlying disease. For patients with upper airway obstruction, who need a continuous positive airway pressure to maintain the patency of the upper airway, "intentional leak" ventilation with CPAP or BiPAP is simple and perfectly appropriate [21,22]. However, BiPAP devices do not generally perform intermittent positive ventilation as well as classical ventilators, especially in term of the maximal delivered pressure above PEEP [23]. Consequently, patients with NMDs or lung disease are often ventilated with non-leak ventilation to ensure adequate alveolar ventilation.

Leak ventilation is also sometime used in tracheotomized patients with plain tracheostomy tubes and who receive assisted ventilation on an intermittent basis; however, "intentional leak" ventilation should not be used for tracheotomized patients who are entirely ventilator-dependent. Non-leak ventilation is usually preferred in those cases [1,12].

The quality of the inspiratory triggers may limit the performance of ventilators. The patient's inspiratory effort may be too low, reducing the ability of the ventilator to detect the onset of inspiration. With a classical pressure trigger, a closed system is mandatory to facilitate the generation of a differential pressure. With an open system (i.e., leak ventilation), triggers based on a flow signal are better than pressure triggers. Indeed, in case of a flow trigger, the ventilator should be able to detect very low flows, especially in young children, who have small TVs. Nevertheless, because of the lack of information disclosed by the manufacturers concerning the principle and algorithms used for the inspiratory trigger, it is difficult to understand why one ventilator seems to exhibit a better trigger than another.

Even though home ventilators are becoming increasingly sophisticated, children with respiratory failure, especially the youngest ones, may develop extreme breathing patterns and low inspiratory effort, which may represent a challenge for a ventilator [21]. The lack of detection of the patient's inspiratory and expiratory effort by the majority of ventilators in infants and young children has been previously observed in the study by Essouri and colleagues [21]. Consequently, home ventilators may not be able to adequately synchronize with the respiratory effort in children [24, 25], and leak compensation may be insufficient for young children. This is explained by the fact that most ventilators have not been specifically developed for pediatric patients. Moreover, most of the home care ventilators are not designed to operate within certain limits (e.g., TV between 50 and 100 mL). Thus, these ventilators may not be suitable for very small infants (< 6 kg) [12].

However, in clinical practice, the clinician has to deal with the available devices. A recent French bench study evaluated the performance of 17 ventilators available for home ventilation with the most common pediatric profiles, namely NMD, upper airway obstruction, and cystic fibrosis [23]. This study confirmed the limitations of the ventilators currently available for home ventilation in children. Indeed, it showed that: (1) no ventilator was perfect and able to adequately ventilate the different patient profiles; (2) ventilator performance was very heterogeneous and depended on the type of trigger and circuit and, most importantly, on the characteristics of the patient; and (3) the sensitivity of the inspiratory triggers of most of the ventilators was insufficient for infants [23]. In particular, the study showed that a total of 12 ventilators had a trigger delay < 150 ms for fewer than two profiles and only one ventilator for three profiles. In all other cases, the trigger was "inappropriate", meaning that ineffective efforts (i.e., the patient was trying to trigger – indicated by an abrupt airway pressure drop simultaneous to a flow decrease–, but the ventilator did not deliver a breath) or auto-triggering (i.e., the ventilator is delivering a mechanical breath without a prior airway pressure decrease, indicating that the ventilator delivers a breath that is not triggered by the patient) were present. Furthermore, most of the home ventilators were unable to cope with additional leaks, resulting in auto-triggering or in the inability to detect the patient's inspiratory effort [23]. Finally, significant differences with regard to the expiratory triggers were also observed in the French study, and some ventilators showed a low pressurization slope, which meant that the ventilator was not able to reach the preset pressure within a minimal time frame [23]. In conclusion, this study underlined the need for a systematic evaluation of all ventilators proposed for home ventilation in children. This evaluation should ideally include an assessment of the quality of the inspiratory and expiratory triggers and of the ability of the ventilator to reach and maintain the preset volume or pressure, as well as to cope with leaks [23].

In clinical practice, the use of a high backup rate, i.e., equivalent to two or three breaths below the patient's spontaneous respiratory frequency, may overcome the problems associated with an inadequate inspiratory trigger. In particular, such a setting is recommended for patients with NMDs [26].

7.7 Noninvasive and Invasive Long-Term Mechanical Ventilation

Interfaces are devices that connect ventilator tubing to the patient, facilitating the entry of pressurized gas into the upper airway. The major difference between invasive and NIV is that with the latter, gas is delivered to the airway through an "interface" rather than an invasive conduit.

NIV represents an interesting alternative to tracheotomy, which is associated with significant morbidity (i.e., tracheomalacia, granuloma formation, soft-tissue infections around the tracheostomy stoma, impaired swallowing) and may impair normal development and, particularly, language development [12,27,28]. Moreover, discomfort and disruption of social and family life are common consequences of patients with a tracheostomy. Finally, although tracheostomized children may be safely discharged home after careful family education and training, home treatment may be difficult or even impracticable for some families [29]. In contrast, home treatment is easier with NIV, which has the main advantage of being noninvasive with the possibility of an "on-demand" use, causing much less discomfort and social life disruption than a tracheotomy.

Several recent studies showed that the majority of children on LTMV are ventilated noninvasively [1,2,7]. While NIV has been used in children and adolescents suffering from severe obstructive sleep apnea syndrome (OSAS) and CRF due to NMDs or lung diseases, more recently it is also being used in younger patients and patients with various diseases associated to severe bilateral facial deformities, such as achondroplasia, craniostenosis, and Down syndrome [30–32]. Moreover, an increasing number of patients may benefit from NIV in the newborn period, such as infants with Pierre Robin syndrome [21,33].

Unfortunately NIV cannot be used with all children because of several reasons [19]: (1) NIV is more difficult to apply in infants and young children than in adults; (2) it requires a minimal respiratory autonomy; and (3) it may be ineffective in patients with severe bulbar involvement with recurrent pulmonary infection or in patients with severe retention of secretions not controlled by noninvasive measures. The inability to tolerate NIV for the amount of time required or ineffective NIV are other causes of NIV failure [12,15].

A recent Italian survey showed that the percentage of noninvasively ventilated patients increased with age, becoming prevalent in those older than 11 years [1]. Moreover, failure to wean from mechanical ventilation and the need for nearly continuous ventilatory assistance were the main causes leading to tracheotomy [1].

It is noteworthy that, in children with SMA type 1 and in other rapidly progressive NMDs, tracheotomy is controversial and an ethical dilemma [8]. Consequently, in these cases, tracheotomy for chronic ventilation is a decision that needs to be carefully discussed if requested by parents.

7.7.1 Noninvasive Long-Term Mechanical Ventilation

The choice of the optimal interface is of paramount importance for the success of NIV, but is also challenging, especially in young children and those with facial deformities. Consequently, the extended use of NIV is limited by the paucity of well-adapted industrial masks for these young children. Furthermore, children may not tolerate NIV in the case of skin injury, pain, discomfort, or air leaks around the mask. Finally, the choice of the interface for NIV is also determined by the ventilatory mode: interfaces with manufactured leaks are used for leak ventilation, while interfaces without manufactured leaks are used for non-leak ventilation.

In chronically, noninvasively ventilated children, five different types of interfaces may be used, i.e., nasal mask, oronasal mask, nasal prongs, mouthpieces, and full-face mask.

7.7.1.1 Nasal Mask
Nasal masks are preferred because they have less anatomical dead space, are less claustrophobic, and allow communication and expectoration more easily than full-face masks [19]. Nasal masks also allow the use of a pacifier in infants, which contributes to the better acceptance of NIV and the reduction of mouth leaks [19].

7.7.1.2 Oronasal Mask
Oronasal masks may be less acceptable to some patients for long-term use because they cover both the nose and mouth, and asphyxiation may be a concern in children who are unable to remove the mask in the event of ventilator malfunction or power failure (i.e., preschool children, children with NMDs, or reduced mobility of the upper limbs) [34]. Furthermore, interference with speech, eating, and expectoration, claustrophobic reactions, and the theoretical risk of aspiration

and rebreathing, are greater with oronasal than nasal masks. Consequently, in children, these interfaces are only used in the case of serious mouth leaks and/or the impossibility to close the mouth during sleep.

7.7.1.3 Nasal Prongs

Nasal prongs are very well tolerated by patients because of the absence of a frontal support, which allows the patient to continue to perform normal daily activities, such as reading, writing, and watching television without much hindrance. Furthermore, Ramirez and colleagues showed that exchanging a nasal mask with nasal prongs was associated with a marked reduction in maxillary retrusion in an adolescent who developed severe facial deformity within a few months after the start of NPPV [34]. However, nasal prongs are often too large for small children [19,34].

7.7.1.4 Mouthpieces

Mouthpieces, held in place by lip seals, are simple and inexpensive interfaces. They may be selectively used in older patients with NMDs [35]. Mouthpiece ventilation is especially useful for daytime ventilatory assistance. The mouthpiece can be placed near the mouth using clamp support, with ventilation supplied by a wheelchair-mounted portable ventilator. For nocturnal use, the mouthpiece is held in place by a strapless bite block. Although mouthpieces have been extensively used in patients with NMDs, they require good cooperation and are difficult to use in young children [19]. In addition, one of their major limitations is the production of large amounts of air leaks, which may compromise NIV efficacy and cause unwanted alarming of the ventilator. Moreover, mouthpieces may stimulate salivation, elicit the gag reflex and, ultimately, cause vomiting. Standard mouthpieces may also produce orthodontic deformities over time [36,37].

7.7.1.5 Full-Face Mask

A total full-face mask (i.e., PerforMax, Respironics, Murrysville, PA, USA) covers the nose, the mouth, and the eyes. By sealing around the perimeter of the face, where patients have less pressure sensitivity and smoother facial contours, it improves comfort, minimizes skin breakdown, and eliminates nasal bridge seal challenges. Although it is usually restricted to the acute setting, the author's experience (Racca and Gregoretti unpublished data) is that some pediatric patients (i.e., > 4 years) can selectively be adapted to this interface without an increase in CO_2 due to the greater dead space (unpublished data).

Custom-made masks may play a major role for infants and children who cannot use industrial masks [38]. Faroux and colleagues [38] found that skin injury was associated with the use of a commercial mask. In their study, the replacement of a commercial mask with a custom-made mask was associated with a reduction in the skin injury score.

A systematic close surveillance of the tolerance of the interface is mandatory in children treated with long-term NIV. First of all, the rapid growth of facial structures in young children is a frequent cause of mask change. Moreover, side effects may be clinically significant in children using NIV, and the interface should be changed or modified at the first sign of intolerance (i.e., discomfort, inefficacy of NIV because of leaks, facial deformity). In these young patients, there is a high risk of skin injury. Faroux and colleagues found that skin injury due to a nasal mask, ranging from transient erythema to permanent skin necrosis, was observed in 53% of the 40 patients during their routine 6-month follow-up [38]. Other facial side effects are facial deformity, such as facial flattening and maxilla retrusion [39,40], caused by the pressure applied by the mask on growing facial structures. The long-term side effects of NIV in children, such as facial flattening or maxillary retrusion, should not be underestimated [38–40]. Thus, systematic close monitoring by a pediatric maxillofacial specialist is mandatory in children treated with long-term NIV [38].

Recently, Ramirez and colleagues reported their study of a large group of infants and children (i.e., 97 children) who were started on long-term NIV [34]. On admission, the most appropriate interface with regard to the patient's underlying disease and ventilatory mode, but also tolerance and comfort, was selected. The patients were tried on the interface with NIV for repeated short periods during the daytime. In infants and children nasal masks were preferred over facial masks, which were only used in the case of serious mouth leaks and/or the impossibility to close the mouth during sleep. In adolescents, nasal prongs were proposed as the first choice in the case of CPAP or BiPAP ventilation. The interface associated with the best tolerance and comfort, defined by the absence of any skin injury, pain, discomfort, and leaks, was selected. All 25 children aged ≤ 2 years, as well as four older children, were fitted with custom-made nasal masks; all other children were fitted with an industrial nasal mask (50%), a facial mask (16%), or nasal prongs (2%). Industrial masks with and without manufactured leaks were used in 33 (34%) and 35 (36%) children, respectively. All patients with obstructive sleep apnea used interfaces with manufactured leaks, whereas all patients with NMD or thoracic scoliosis used interfaces without manufactured leaks. Both types of interfaces were used in patients with lung disease. It is noteworthy that, in this study, even after a careful selection of the most appropriate interface by an experienced NIV and maxillofacial team, discomfort and side effects occurred in as many as 21% of the patients, justifying systematic and close monitoring of the NIV interface. The interface had to be changed in 20 patients because of discomfort (n = 16), leaks (n = 4), facial growth (n = 3), skin injury (n = 2), or change of the ventilatory mode (n = 2). A second or third mask change was necessary in nine and four patients, respectively [34].

7.7.2 Long-Term Mechanical Ventilation via Tracheostomy

Generally, small, plain tracheostomy tubes should be used [12]. These prevent tracheomalacia, and a large leak around the tracheostomy facilitates speech. Disposable plastic tracheostomy tubes under size 4 do not have an inner cannula and thus should be changed on a regular basis at home.

The majority of tracheostomized children are ventilated with VTV [1,12]. Ventilator-assisted children generally have uncuffed plain tracheostomies [1,12]. As a consequence, a portion of the TV delivered by the ventilator is leaked around the tracheostomy tube through the native airway. Because, in some children, this leak is relatively constant, a higher TV (e.g., 10–15 mL/kg) can be used to compensate the leak so that adequate ventilation can be achieved [12]. Otherwise, the tracheostomy leak can be compensated by using the ventilator in a pressure modality; alternatively, partially inflated cuffed tracheostomy tubes may be used [12].

Most children require tracheostomy tube changes in the range of weekly to monthly. However, frequency should depend on individual factors [12]. For example, changes may need to be more frequent during respiratory infections or in patients with increased tracheal secretions.

All caregivers, whether they are performing routine tracheostomy tube changes or not, should learn the technique in the event that an emergency or unexpected tracheostomy tube change is required. A second sterile tracheostomy tube must always be available in case of accidental decannulation. In addition, a tracheostomy tube with an external diameter smaller than the one in place should be available for an emergency maneuver (e.g., when the tracheostomy tube cannot be easily replaced) [12].

7.8 Additional Equipment for Pediatric Home Ventilation

7.8.1 Need for an Alternate Power Supply for the Ventilator

Supplemental batteries are indicated for home use when power failures are common, when patients may suffer adverse consequences during even brief power outages, and in cases where mobility is important [12]. In fact, a child who requires continuous ventilation should have a battery, not only to allow mobility in a wheelchair, but also to avoid catastrophic consequences in the event of a power failure. These batteries must be checked regularly to ensure proper function. Children requiring only nocturnal mechanical ventilation may not need a battery.

Backup generators may be useful in remote areas where power failures may be prolonged [12].

7.8.2 Backup Ventilators

For children who have < 4 consecutive hours of free time from the ventilator, a backup ventilator is necessary because these children cannot tolerate the length of time that may be required for the provider to bring a functioning ventilator to the patient. Furthermore, backup ventilators are also necessary for children who live at a great distance from medical care or from their home providers [12].

Both ventilators should be used alternatively to assure that both remain functional.

7.8.3 Humidifiers

All patients receiving continuous mechanical ventilation through tracheostomy require that the inspired gas is warmed and humidified to prevent drying and thickening of tracheobronchial secretions. Humidifiers may be of the water reservoir type (bubble through or passover) or of the heat and moisture exchange type (artificial nose). Since water reservoir type humidifiers are more effective, they are recommended for all tracheostomized patients, except during short periods away from home [12]. During these short periods (< 12 h) away from the care setting, heat and moisture exchangers are preferred.

Humidifiers are not required in many patients using nasal or face mask ventilation, but are needed for patients in dry climates or during the winter months, or for patients using mouthpiece ventilation. A heat and moisture exchanger is not recommended because there is a large volume of gas moving through the device. In addition, these should be avoided with BiPAP devices because they add resistance and may alter the inspiratory and expiratory pressures [12].

7.8.4 Suction Machines and Suction Catheters

All patients receiving mechanical ventilation through tracheostomy require a portable suction machine. They should be electronically and battery-powered [12]. Although a sterile technique is mandatory in acute and intermediate care facilities as well as in long-term skilled nursing facilities, suctioning at home should be performed using a clean technique, with maintenance of standard precautions. In this technique, nondisposable suction catheters can be cleaned and reused [12].

7.8.5 Oxygen Therapy and Pulse Oximeter

The goal of home oxygen therapy is to maintain a sufficient PaO_2 to prevent the cardiovascular or central nervous system complications of hypoxia while optimizing the child's lifestyle and rehabilitative potential. This generally requires a PaO_2 > 65 mmHg (> 95% SpO_2 of hemoglobin) at sea level [12]. Oxygen should also be used for emergency rescue maneuvers.

If additional oxygen is required in ventilator-dependent children, liquid O_2 tanks should be used. Small portable cylinders allow for mobility of the oxygen-dependent child.

Because PaO_2 varies considerably with sleep, feeding, and physical activity, especially in infants and small children, continuous noninvasive monitoring techniques (i.e., pulse oximeter) should be used to assess the adequacy of oxygenation during periods of sleep, wakefulness, feeding, and physical activity.

Pulse oximeters should also be used in children with NMDs. Indeed, Bach and colleagues [41,42] described a regimen for managing acute-on-chronic neuromuscular respiratory failure at home, which includes the use of a pulse oximeter. The patient receives 24-h mechanical ventilation during exacerbation; pulse oximetry is monitored continuously and when SpO_2 on room air falls below 95%, secretions are aggressively removed with mechanical in-exsufflation (MI-E) until SpO_2 returns to 95%.

7.8.6 Monitoring

For most patients, a pulse oximeter is sufficient for adequate home monitoring. Capnography may be useful in selected patients [12].

7.8.7 Self-Inflating Resuscitation Bag

All patients receiving mechanical ventilation through tracheostomy require a self-inflating resuscitation bag with mask.

7.9 Noninvasive Aids for Secretion Clearance

NIV should be combined with airway clearance techniques for all patients with weakened expiratory muscles who have excessive secretions [8,9,12]. Airway clearance is very important in the chronic management of all patients with NMD. Indeed, effective airway clearance is critical for patients to prevent atelectasis and pneumonia. Ineffective airway clearance can hasten the onset of respiratory failure and death, whereas early intervention to improve airway clearance can prevent hospitalization and reduce the incidence of pneumonia [8,9,12].

Assessment of the patient's ability to clear secretions is done primarily by measuring peak cough flow (PCF). PCF can be obtained with a simple peak flow meter connected to a fitted mask while asking the child to cough. PCFs of 160–270 L/min have been described as acceptable levels to clear the airway in adults and adolescents. Below this point, patients are more susceptible to infection and respiratory failure [9,15]. Children with NMDs may be too weak or too young to perform this measurement. Therefore, the most useful evaluation of respiratory muscle function may be observation of cough ability [8].

Various techniques have been developed to overcome ineffective cough in patients with neuromuscular weakness. Noninvasive techniques for secretion clearance include manually assisted coughing and mechanical insufflator-exsufflator (MI-E). MI-E is usually employed when manually assisted coughing is inadequate. MI-E is contraindicated in patients with bullous emphysema or other disorders associated with a predisposition to barotraumas [12]. Oral suctioning can assist in managing secretions after assisted coughing [8]. Home pulse oximetry is useful to monitor the effectiveness of airway clearance during respiratory illnesses. Caregivers should learn how to assist coughing in all patients with ineffective cough.

7.10   Home Discharge and Regular Follow-Up

Since discharging a ventilator-dependent child to home imposes a significant burden on the family, the physician should inform patient and family of such a burden, as well as the benefits of home LTMV.

Before the patient's home discharge, all caregivers must be trained and need to demonstrate competency in all the care procedures the patient will require. In particular, training should include the correct use of equipment and supplies. Moreover, parents of a LTMV child should be trained to recognize and correct the most common problems, such as tube dislocation or tube obstruction.

The planning of home LTMV requires communication between territorial and hospital structures. In particular, the general practitioner and local health service must be involved. Furthermore, nurses, physiotherapists, and speech therapists from territorial structures may be required at home.

Before children are discharged home, the equipment and supplies required for the continuation of ventilator assistance must be provided by the local health service. Furthermore, equipment companies should provide equipment maintenance and help in case of malfunction.

A written comprehensive management plan, covering both respiratory and other medical care, should be developed before discharge (Table 7.3). This plan should be based on the physician's instructions and used by the caregivers and ancillary personnel to guide them in the daily care of the child.

Finally, a scheduled regular follow-up program should be an essential element of the home discharge. Follow-up visits are justified and medically necessary for the evaluation of changes in clinical status and for care plan modifications when they are necessary. The patient in a stable condition should be seen by their physician, who should be experienced in the management of LTMV at appropriate intervals. More frequent visits are required immediately following home transfer and as warranted by the patient's medical condition. The ventilator-assisted patient can be transported to the physician's office.

7.11   Conclusions

Larger prospective studies are warranted to determine:
1. the criteria to initiate LTMV according to the patient's age and underlying disease;
2. the long-term benefits (i.e., increase in survival, stabilization in the decline in lung function and respiratory muscle performance);
3. whether LTMV may improve the child's and family's quality of life; and
4. the type of equipment and the specific ventilator settings that should be chosen.

Table 7.3 Care plan checklist

Mechanical ventilator, active humidifier, and ventilator circuit information:
- detailed description of circuits
- detailed description of ventilator power source
- instructions for cleaning and assembling the ventilator
- specific times on and off the ventilator
- description of mode of ventilation
- desired pressure and TV ranges
- description of alarms
- range of pulse oximetry
- equipment company phone number for help in case of ventilator malfunction

Name, size, and type of noninvasive interface (for noninvasive ventilatory support only)

Instructions for the care of the noninvasive interface (for noninvasive ventilatory support only)
- instructions for cleaning and assembling the interface
- instructions for reducing the risk of skin breakdown (e.g., barrier dressing, such as hydro- colloid sheet)
- instructions for securing the mask (e.g., avoid air leaks although allowing enough space to pass two fingers under the head strap)

Name, size, and type (cuffed or uncuffed, double or single cannula, fenestrated or not fenestrated) **of artificial airway** (for invasive ventilatory support only)

Instructions for the care of the artificial airway (for invasive ventilatory support only)
- conditions for inflation/deflation, if appropriate
- airway care plan (tube changes, cleaning, problem-solving)
- airway suctioning (detailed description of sterile technique for suctioning)
- medications

Description of self-inflating resuscitation bag use (for invasive ventilatory support only)

Adjunctive techniques
- pulse oximeter use
- oxygen therapy use, if appropriate
- secretion clearance devices use, if appropriate
- regimen for managing acute-on-chronic respiratory failure at home
- aerosol (bronchodilator), if appropriate
- chest physiotherapy, if appropriate

Notification of local emergency care facilities

Equipment and supplies for LTMV (e.g., interfaces or tracheostomy tube, ventilator circuits, and so on) **prescribed and provided at home**

First follow-up program scheduled

Documentation of the education of caregivers

Other medical care

LTMV long-term mechanical ventilation, *TV* tidal volume

References

1. Racca, F, Bonati M, Del Sorbo L et al (2011) Invasive and non-invasive long-term mechanical ventilation in Italian children. Minerva Anestesiol 77(9):892-901
2. Racca, F, Berta G, Sequi M et al (2011) Long-term home ventilation of children in Italy: a national survey. Pediatr Pulmonol 46(6):566-572
3. Graham, RJ, Fleegler E W, Robinson WM (2007) Chronic ventilator need in the community: a 2005 pediatric census of Massachusetts. Pediatrics 119(6):e1280-e1287
4. Gowans M, Keenan HT, Bratton SL (2007) The population prevalence of children receiving invasive home ventilation in Utah. Pediatr Pulmonol 42(3):231-236
5. Edwards EA, Hsiao K, Nixon GM (2005) Paediatric home ventilatory support: the Auckland experience. J Paediatr Child Health 41(12):652-658
6. Jardine E, O'Toole M, Paton JY et al (1999) Current status of long term ventilation of children in the United Kingdom: questionnaire survey. BMJ 318(7179):295-299
7. Wallis C, Paton JY, Beaton S et al (2011) Children on long-term ventilatory support: 10 years of progress. Arch Dis Child 96(11):998-1002
8. Wang CH, Finkel RS, Bertini ES et al (2007) Consensus statement for standard of care in spinal muscular atrophy. J Child Neurol 22(8):1027-1049
9. Finder JD, Birnkrant D, Carl J et al (2004) Respiratory care of the patient with Duchenne muscular dystrophy: ATS consensus statement. Am J Respir Crit Care Med 170(4):456-465
10. Annane D, Orlikowski D, Chevret S et al (2007) Nocturnal mechanical ventilation for chronic hypoventilation in patients with neuromuscular and chest wall disorders. Cochrane Database Syst Rev (4):CD001941
11. Katz S, Selvadurai H, Keilty K et al (2004) Outcome of non-invasive positive pressure ventilation in paediatric neuromuscular disease. Arch Dis Child 89(2):121-124
12. Make BJ, Hill NS, Goldberg AI et al (1998) Mechanical ventilation beyond the intensive care unit. Report of a consensus conference of the American College of Chest Physicians. Chest 113(5 Suppl):S289-S344
13. Nørregaard O (2008) NIV: indication in case of acute respiratory failure in children
14. White DP, Douglas NJ, Pickett CK et al (1983) Sleep deprivation and the control of ventilation. Am Rev Respir Dis 128(6):984-986
15. Wang CH, Bonnemann CG, Rutkowski A et al (2010) Consensus statement on standard of care for congenital muscular dystrophies. J Child Neurol 25(12):1559-1581
16. Bushby K, Finkel R, Birnkrant DJ et al (2010) Diagnosis and management of Duchenne muscular dystrophy, part 2: implementation of multidisciplinary care. Lancet Neurol 9(2):177-189
17. Chatwin M, Bush A, Simonds AK (2011) Outcome of goal-directed non-invasive ventilation and mechanical insufflation/exsufflation in spinal muscular atrophy type I. Arch Dis Child 96(5):426-432
18. Fauroux B (2011) Why, when and how to propose noninvasive ventilation in cystic fibrosis? Minerva Anestesiol 77(11):1108-1114
19. Fauroux BAG, Lofaso F (2008) NIV and chronic respiratory failure in children, Eur Respir Mon
20. Brochard L, Pluskwa F, Lemaire F (1987) Improved efficacy of spontaneous breathing with inspiratory pressure support. Am Rev Respir Dis 136(2):411-415
21. Essouri S, Nicot F, Clement A et al (2005) "Noninvasive positive pressure ventilation in infants with upper airway obstruction: comparison of continuous and bilevel positive pressure" Intensive Care Med 31(4):574-580
22. Marcus CL, Rosen G, Ward SL et al (2006) Adherence to and effectiveness of positive airway pressure therapy in children with obstructive sleep apnea. Pediatrics 117(3):e442-e451
23. Fauroux B, Leroux K, Desmarais G et al (2008) Performance of ventilators for noninvasive positive-pressure ventilation in children. Eur Respir J 31(6):1300-1307
24. Fauroux B, Louis B, Hart N et al (2004) The effect of back-up rate during non-invasive ventilation in young patients with cystic fibrosis. Intensive Care Med 30(4):673-681

25. Fauroux B, Nicot F, Essouri S et al (2004) Setting of noninvasive pressure support in young patients with cystic fibrosis. Eur Respir J 24(4):624-630
26. (1999) Clinical indications for noninvasive positive pressure ventilation in chronic respiratory failure due to restrictive lung disease, COPD, and nocturnal hypoventilation – a consensus conference report. Chest 116:521-534
27. Dubey SP, Garap JP (1999) Paediatric tracheostomy: an analysis of 40 cases. J Laryngol Otol 113(7):645-651
28. Wetmore RF, Marsh RR, Thompson ME et al (1999) Pediatric tracheostomy: a changing procedure? Ann Otol Rhinol Laryngol 108(7 Pt 1):695-699
29. Ruben RJ, Newton L, Jornsay D et al (1982) Home care of the pediatric patient with a tracheotomy. Ann Otol Rhinol Laryngol 91(6 Pt 1):633-640
30. Waters KA, Everett F, Sillence DO et al (1995) Treatment of obstructive sleep apnea in achondroplasia: evaluation of sleep, breathing, and somatosensory-evoked potentials. Am J Med Genet 59(4):460-466
31. Ottonello G, Villa G, Moscatelli A et al (2007) Noninvasive ventilation in a child affected by achondroplasia respiratory difficulty syndrome. Paediatr Anaesth 17(1):75-79
32. Anzai Y, Ohya T, Yanagi K (2006) Treatment of sleep apnea syndrome in a Down syndrome patient with behavioral problems by noninvasive positive pressure ventilation: a successful case report. No To Hattatsu 38(1):32-36
33. Leboulanger N, Picard A, Soupre V et al (2010) Physiologic and clinical benefits of noninvasive ventilation in infants with Pierre Robin sequence. Pediatrics 126(5):e1056-e1063
34. Ramirez A, Delord V, Khirani S et al (2012) Interfaces for long-term noninvasive positive pressure ventilation in children. Intensive Care Med 38(4):655-662
35. Niranjan V, Bach JR (1998) Noninvasive management of pediatric neuromuscular ventilatory failure. Crit Care Med 26(12):2061-2065
36. Nava S, Navalesi P, Gregoretti C (2009) Interfaces and humidification for noninvasive mechanical ventilation. Respir Care 54(1):71-84
37. Toussaint M, Steens M, Wasteels G et al (2006) Diurnal ventilation via mouthpiece: survival in end-stage Duchenne patients. Eur Respir J 28(3):549-555
38. Fauroux B, Lavis JF, Nicot F et al (2005) Facial side effects during noninvasive positive pressure ventilation in children. Intensive Care Med 31(7):965-969
39. Li KK, Riley RW, Guilleminault C (2000) An unreported risk in the use of home nasal continuous positive airway pressure and home nasal ventilation in children: mid-face hypoplasia. Chest 117(3):916-918
40. Villa MP, Pagani J, Ambrosio R et al (2002) Mid-face hypoplasia after long-term nasal ventilation. Am J Respir Crit Care Med 166(8):1142-1143
41. Tzeng AC, Bach JR (2000) Prevention of pulmonary morbidity for patients with neuromuscular disease. Chest 118(5):1390-1396
42. Bach JR, Rajaraman R, Ballanger F et al (1998) Neuromuscular ventilatory insufficiency: effect of home mechanical ventilator use v oxygen therapy on pneumonia and hospitalization rates. Am J Phys Med Rehabil 77(1):8-19

Part II

Anesthesia and Perioperative Medicine

Anesthesia and Perioperative Medicine

8

Adrian T. Bosenberg

8.1 Introduction

The perioperative preparation of children presenting for surgery aims to identify medical problems that influence the outcome and to institute management strategies to reduce those problems. Respiratory complications remain the most significant cause of morbidity and mortality in modern pediatric anesthesia [1]. Some common medical problems that are encountered in daily clinical practice include the child with an upper respiratory tract infection (URTI), the child with allergies, and the child with asthma. The ideal management of these problems invokes discussion almost on a daily basis because the guidelines are not clear-cut, and the risks may be significant and even potentially life-threatening, particularly when managed incorrectly. Comorbidity involving any combination of these problems significantly increases the risk [2–8].

8.2 Upper Respiratory Tract Infections

Most young children have frequent URTIs. They present with a spectrum of signs and symptoms depending on the acuteness of the illness. It stands to reason that at some point children will present for surgery with an acute infection or soon after a recent URTI. The dilemma as to whether to cancel, proceed, or postpone elective surgery has been a source of debate for many years [2–8]. All too often, particularly in short stay surgery, this decision is left to the anesthesiologist, who is pressured to make last-minute decisions by the family, the surgeon, or even by

A.T. Bosenberg (✉)
Department Anesthesiology and Pain Management
Faculty of Health Sciences, University of Washington, Seattle Children's Hospital
Seattle, USA
e-mail: adrian.bosenberg@seattlechildrens.org

M. Astuto (ed.) *Pediatric Anesthesia, Intensive Care and Pain: Standardization in Clinical Practice*. Anesthesia, Intensive Care and Pain in Neonates and Children
DOI: 10.1007/978-88-470-2685-8_8, © Springer-Verlag Italia 2013

the hospital management. Late cancelations can be very disruptive to the surgical schedule.

In reviewing the literature, there is little uniformity or single definition of an URTI that can be universally applied. Many researchers select certain surgical procedures and times of the year to ensure maximal enrollment for their study. Severe cases are excluded. Definitions vary from one publication to the next, but essentially children fall into three categories [2–8]. First, there are those who present with a fever, malaise, rhinorrhea (clear or purulent), sore or scratchy throat, sneezing, nasal congestion, productive cough, and chest signs and who are clearly not well. This group is straightforward and surgery *should be canceled* unless the procedure is an emergency. This group is excluded from most studies.

The second group develop symptoms a day or two before the elective procedure, the parents call the surgeon or anesthesiologist the night before, surgery is canceled and they are rescheduled in *2 weeks*, and the child returns with minimal or no symptoms. Alternatively, a conversation with the parents clarifies the severity of the symptoms and a decision is made to re-evaluate the child on the morning of surgery.

The majority of children fall into the third category, i.e., those who have had an URTI with symptoms for days or even weeks, and who are stable or improving. Most studies exclude the first and second group and only include those with mild URTI symptoms.

Although an URTI implies an upper airway problem, the upper and lower airways are always involved to a variable degree. Viral infections damage the ciliary apparatus and mucosal epithelium exposing the underlying nerve endings. Consequently, the airway is sensitized to the irritant effect of the inhalational agents and secretions. Airway smooth muscle activity is enhanced. In addition, ventilation-perfusion mismatch occurs, closing volume increases, and there is a reduction in functional residual capacity. Although the clinical symptoms resolve, usually within 2 weeks, airway irritability may persist for up to 6–8 weeks. It is the severity of these subclinical changes that ultimately influences the decision to defer surgery [3].

Airway-related events, the most common adverse anesthetic problem, include airway obstruction, bronchospasm, laryngospasm, breath holding, post-extubation croup, cough, desaturation, and bradycardia [3–5], and anecdotal reports of atelectasis, pneumonia, and even death [9–12]. Factors that have been shown to increase the risk of these respiratory events include more symptomatic children (nasal congestion, copious secretions), airway instrumentation in children under 5 years, surgery involving the airway, a history of reactive airways or snoring, prematurity, parental confirmation of the presence of an URTI, and passive smoking [3,5]. Infants under 6 months are at greatest risk.

Viral myocarditis, a particularly difficult clinical diagnosis, has been described in a number of sudden deaths under anesthesia [9–12]. Although rare, unsuspected myocarditis remains a major concern in the child with symptoms of a "cold."

When making a preoperative assessment, it is important to exclude symptoms that are related to an allergy (usually seasonal) or whether they are the prodromal symptoms of an infectious disease (e.g., measles, mumps, chicken pox, rubella, meningococcal infection) that may put other patients or staff at risk. Some syndromic children may have a persistent mucopurulent rhinitis (Down syndrome, Hurler/Hunter syndrome, cleft palate, patent ductus arteriosus) that may influence the decision. In these children, rhinitis is common and it is important to establish whether there has been a change in the character of the secretions suggesting an acute-on-chronic infection. Unilateral rhinorrhea suggests unilateral nasal obstruction (foreign body, polyp).

When is it safe to proceed? The ideal time to reschedule surgery is far from settled. Airway hypersensitivity and reactivity persists for up to 6 weeks, particularly if the lower airway is involved. Some authors suggest that the lower airways are always involved! Children may have between three and eight URTIs per annum. It is conceivable that if surgery is delayed for 4–6 weeks after each episode, there may be only a small window when the child is asymptomatic and "fit" for surgery if this guideline is applied.

Tait and colleagues [4] showed that the incidence of easily treatable airway complications was similar in the acutely symptomatic to those who had symptoms for 4 weeks. In this study [4], which included 1,078 children (1 month-18 years) with *mild* URTI symptoms, they showed that children who presented for elective surgery with a recent URTI (within 4 weeks) fared as well as those with acute symptoms. They concluded that with careful airway management most of these children can undergo elective procedures without increased morbidity or long-term sequelae. There was no statistically significant difference in the incidence of laryngospasm or bronchospasm in the acute or recent URTI with mild symptoms compared to the asymptomatic children. Although these children have an increased risk of adverse respiratory events (coughing, breath holding, desaturation), these are easily treatable by experienced anesthesiologists.

Schreiner and colleagues [6] showed that nearly 2,000 cases would have had to be canceled to prevent 15 cases of laryngospasm in experienced hands. Delaying or canceling the procedure does not significantly alter the incidence of adverse respiratory events. Little is gained except to create an inconvenience for the family and all concerned to prevent an easily treatable problem occurring in the minority of patients.

Predicting which child with URTI is likely to have an adverse event has recently been studied [13]. Adverse respiratory events occurred when children were symptomatic or were symptomatic less than 2 weeks before the procedure, whereas symptoms that were present 2–4 weeks prior lowered the risk. Other risk factors included a family history of atopy, asthma, and passive smoking.

The management of adverse respiratory events should evolve according to the particular circumstances, the cause, the drugs and equipment available, and the child's underlying condition. Most events respond to simple maneuvers, such as continuous positive airway pressure support, and simple therapeutic measures. Bronchodilators (best given intravenously), suxamethonium 1 mg/kg, lidocaine 1 mg/kg, endotracheal intubation, and short-term ventilation should all be considered and used as indicated. Deepening the anesthesia without compromising the child may also bring resolution.

The ideal anesthetic is also a matter of debate. Differences in study design and a lack of uniformity regarding the types and surgical procedures and the duration thereof, the types of airway instrumentation, and the choice of anesthetic for the child with an URTI has provided no answers. Anesthetic management should aim to reduce stimulation of a potentially irritable airway. Propofol has major advantages over other agents. Isoflurane and desflurane both cause significant airway irritability and should be avoided. Any airway instrumentation is associated with more adverse respiratory events [6,13,14]. A face mask is considered the method of choice whenever possible [3,5,14]. A laryngeal mask airway [LMA] has fewer complications [3,14] than endotracheal intubation which, in some studies, is associated with an 11-fold increase in adverse events [6]. The risk of deep extubation is no different from awake extubation.

In today's economic climate and managed health-care environment, other factors come into the equation. These include the distance traveled to the hospital, whether the parents have taken special leave, the attitude of the family, the number of previous cancelations and the experience of the anesthesiologist. The impact of cancelation on the family can be substantial. Disruption of the operating schedule and the cost of staffing an operating room that goes unused are further considerations. These should not directly influence the decision – but realistically they often do! Ultimately, the child's safety should be the primary consideration.

8.3   Allergy

Parents frequently indicate that their children have multiple drug allergies, though often these have not been validated. Parents confuse side effects with a true allergy. Potential allergic cross-reactivity between drugs and foods are frequently considered perioperative risk factors that need to be addressed. Allergenic cross-reactivity is a property defined by individual antibodies to other allergens with structural similarity and can be seen in families of drugs or agents used during the perioperative period. "Multiple drug allergy syndrome" or "multiple drug hypersensitivity" is a clinical condition characterized by the propensity to react to chemically unrelated drugs, mainly antibiotics [15]. In most cases, the syndrome presents as acute urticaria, angioedema, or both after administration of the allergenic compounds [15].

Immediate allergic hypersensitivity reactions are triggered by specific immunological mechanisms mediated by antibodies [usually immunoglobulin E (IgE) isotype] and can lead to life-threatening symptoms [16]. The main risk factor for anaphylaxis is a previous uninvestigated severe immediate hypersensitivity reaction during the perioperative period. Neuromuscular blocking agents and antibiotics are the most common triggers. If possible, a history of drug-induced anaphylaxis should be confirmed by an appropriate evaluation wherever possible [16–20].

Many food allergies (egg, soy, peanut, seafood/fish, shellfish) are often mistakenly considered a contraindication to some medications, although the evidence for this is lacking. Many false assumptions about drug allergies are mostly based on anecdotal case reports. The evidence suggests that egg-allergic, soy-allergic, or peanut-allergic patients are not more likely to develop anaphylaxis when exposed to propofol. Egg allergy is most common during childhood and is usually outgrown by adulthood [21]. Egg-allergic patients generally demonstrate immediate hypersensitivity to proteins from egg white (ovomucoid, ovalbumin), whereas lecithin, which is not the allergenic determinant, is found in the egg yolk. Propofol is marketed in an oil-in-water emulsion using soybean oil (10%) and egg lecithin (1.2%) as the emulsifying agents. The documented anaphylactic reactions are caused by the isopropyl or phenol groups in propofol rather than the lipid vehicle [22,23]. There is therefore little or no reason to contraindicate propofol in egg-allergic patients.

There is also little or no reason to contraindicate propofol in children with soy allergy or peanut allergy either. Soy allergy is an early-onset food allergy affecting approximately 0.4% of children. Most children develop tolerance by late childhood [24]. Refined soybean oil, such as that present in propofol, is safe for people with soy allergy because the allergenic proteins are removed during the refining process. Soy and peanuts are both leguminous plants and thus any cross-reactivity should not necessitate avoiding propofol.

Shellfish (crustaceans, mollusks) or fish are among the most common foods provoking severe anaphylaxis [25]. The major allergen in fish is the muscle protein parvalbumin, while tropomyosin is the major allergen in crustaceans. Shellfish allergens do not cross-react with fish allergens. Because the allergenic determinants for shellfish and fish are muscle proteins and not other components, such as iodine, there is no reason to modify the anesthetic protocol in cases of shellfish-allergic or fish-allergic patients. There is no cross-reactivity among iodinated contrast agents, povidone-iodine or seafood, as the allergenic determinant is not iodine for any of them. The only contraindication to povidone-iodine is a previous documented hypersensitivity reaction. Although the precise allergenic agent in povidone-iodine has not been elucidated, it is not the iodine atom [26].

8.4 Asthma

Asthma is a disorder that presents with a spectrum of symptoms, including airway obstruction, inflammation, and hyperresponsiveness. It is a chronic inflammatory disorder of the airways that in susceptible individuals may cause recurrent episodes of coughing (particularly at night or in the early morning), wheezing, shortness of breath, and chest tightness. These episodes are usually associated with widespread but variable airflow obstruction that is often reversible either spontaneously or with treatment.

Worldwide, particularly in industrialized countries, asthma seems to be on the increase. It is estimated that up to 300 million people are affected and asthma is implicated in one of every 250 deaths. The prevalence of asthma in children based on a previous diagnosis of asthma and more than one asthma attack during the previous year is 5.5%. Contributing factors that predispose to the development and severity of asthma include genetic predisposition, a history of atopy, exposure to airborne allergens (exposure and sensitivity to house-dust mite), and a history of viral respiratory infections (commonly respiratory syncytial virus or rhinovirus) [29]. Asthma-triggering agents include respiratory infections, inhalants (animal fur, house-dust mites, mold, or pollens), irritants (cigarette smoke), temperature changes (cold air), exercise, and anxiety. The Expert Panel Report 3 of the National Asthma Education and Prevention Program categorizes asthmatics into groups based on the severity of their disease [27].

Asthma ultimately represents a dynamic interaction between host and environmental factors. The immunological-inflammatory pathways involved in the pathogenesis of asthma are complex and include lymphocytes, IgE, eosinophils, neutrophils, mast cells, leukotrienes, and cytokines. These pathways are triggered and modified by extrinsic and environmental factors such as the aforementioned triggers.

The asthmatic child, even when asymptomatic, is at risk of perioperative morbidity (bronchospasm, anaphylaxis), which may progress to mortality if not recognized or poorly managed. This is particularly true if exposed to allergens or other triggering agents during anesthesia.

Especially important in the preoperative evaluation is assessment of disease severity and how well asthma symptoms are currently being controlled. The mainstay of treatment is inhaled β_2-adrenergic agonists (quick- or long-acting) by metered-dose inhalers [28]. The long-acting agents do not suppress inflammation and should not be used without anti-inflammatory treatment for the control of asthma. Inhaled and parenteral corticosteroids are the cornerstone of therapy to stabilize and improve persistent asthma. Leukotriene modifiers inhibit the leukotriene pathway, a mediator of bronchoconstriction. Evidence of their beneficial effect on inflammation is conflicting and they are not useful in acute treatment [28].

Information regarding medication, including oral steroid use, emergency visits, or admissions to the hospital that included intravenous infusions or intubation should be obtained. All give an indication as to the severity of the disease. The previous anesthetic history, presence of known allergies, cough or sputum production, and level of activity should also be assessed. Asthmatics with "atopy" are particularly predisposed to have allergic reactions. The anesthesiologist should be prepared for the possibility of an anaphylactic reaction to allergens in the operating room, such as antibiotics, muscle relaxants, or latex.

When asthma is well controlled, it probably confers no additional risk of perioperative complications; when it is poorly controlled, it almost always does [30]. Prior to elective procedures, optimal control of symptoms should be achieved. If not well controlled, the child should be deferred for additional therapy, which may need to include a short course of oral steroids. Oral prednisone or dexamethasone may be needed [29,30]. Patients with asthma should not have elective surgery during an acute viral respiratory infection since the risk of laryngospasm and bronchospasm is high.

On the day of surgery, patients with asthma should continue their medications as usual. Inhaled β_2-adrenergic agonists should be given 1–2 h prior to surgery. Premedication is usually indicated (oral midazolam, 0.5–1 mg/kg) since anxiety may precipitate an acute episode. Systemic corticosteroids use in the previous 6 months is an indication for "stress dose" coverage to avoid adrenal crisis. High-dose inhaled corticosteroids use may also indicate perioperative stress dose coverage in certain patients.

The anesthetic plan should provide a balance between suppression and avoidance of bronchospasm, with the usual goals of patient safety, comfort, and a quiet surgical field. Drugs that release histamine from mast cells should be avoided. These include thiopentone, many muscle relaxants (atracurium besylate, tubocurarine, mivacurium chloride), and analgesics (morphine). Ketamine is ideal since it produces smooth muscle relaxation and bronchodilation both directly and via the release of catecholamines. Propofol causes profound depression of airway reflexes and when compared to thiopentone there is a significantly lower incidence of wheezing following intubation [31]. The α_2-adrenergic receptor agonist dexmedetomidine has a favorable profile, including anxiolysis, sympatholysis, and drying of secretions without respiratory depression [26], but it is still "off label".

Airway instrumentation under a light level of anesthesia should be avoided. Avoiding intubation by using a mask or LMA for appropriate cases is optimal. An inhaled β_2-adrenergic agonist immediately prior to induction may decrease the risk of bronchospasm that can occur with intubation [32]. Topical local anesthesia (lidocaine 5 mg/kg maximum) is also useful as it blunts the sensory loop of the reflex arc, thus preventing reflex bronchoconstriction. An aerosol spray, which contains a propellant in addition to lidocaine, however, may trigger airway reactivity. A squirt of lidocaine directed to the upper airway from a syringe, or intravenous lidocaine, is preferable.

Sevoflurane is the agent of choice for inhalational induction for a variety of reasons. Sevoflurane has a positive bronchodilating effect, and a lower incidence of laryngospasm and cardiac dysrhythmias compared to halothane, isoflurane, or other volatile anesthetics. Propofol infusion can also be used for maintenance of anesthesia. Desflurane, an airway irritant, can also cause an elevation in airway resistance in children with airway susceptibility and should not be used.

Intraoperatively, bronchospasm can be provoked by laryngoscopy, tracheal intubation, airway suctioning, cold inspired gases, and tracheal extubation. Airway tone is increased by vagal stimulation caused by endoscopy, and by peritoneal or visceral stretch [26]. Inhalation agents and gases should be humidified to prevent inspissation of the already thick secretions. Tracheal suctioning should be performed only when the child is deeply anesthetized or when there is topical anesthesia. The mode of ventilation should be at low inflating pressures with a prolonged expiratory time. Deep extubation potentially avoids the risk of bronchospasm from coughing on the endotracheal tube. Reversal of neuromuscular blockade with neostigmine does not cause bronchospasm if atropine or glycopyrrolate are administered concurrently.

With regard to postoperative analgesia, regional anesthetic techniques are useful. There is concern with regard to the use of nonsteroidal anti-inflammatory drugs (NSAIDs). Despite the fact that many asthmatics have used ibuprofen without problems, a recent meta-analysis suggests that NSAIDs should be avoided in those who have a history of an adverse response to a nonsteroidal drug and in those who have not been previously exposed to a nonsteroidal drug [33].

8.5 Conclusions

In the preoperative assessment of children with URTIs or asthma, the anesthesiologist should focus on signs and symptoms that quantify respiratory status. Parents are useful barometers of their child's condition, which changes from baseline on a day-to-day basis. Children with coexisting pulmonary disease, particularly reactive airway disease, and infants under 6 months of age with an active URTI are at greater risk. Allergies (food or drug) may present additional confounders.

The final decision to proceed with surgery should rest with the individual anesthesiologist and their ability, experience, and comfort level in managing predictable complications in a child with URTI or asthma. Clearly, those with more experience may be prepared to proceed with younger patients with or without additional pathology while others with less experience may not. Whatever the decision, the child's safety remains paramount!

References

1. Bhananker SM, Ramamoorthy C, Geiduschek JM et al (2007) Anesthesia-related cardiac arrest in children: update from the Pediatric Perioperative Cardiac Arrest Registry. Anesth Analg 105:344-350
2. Cote C (2001) The upper respiratory tract infection (URI) dilemma. Fear of complication or litigation. Anesthesiology 95:283-285
3. Ellwood T, Bailey K (2005) The pediatric patient and upper respiratory tract infections. Best Pract Res Clin Anaesth 19:35-46
4. Tait AR, Malviya S, Voepel-Lewis T et al (2001) Risk factors for perioperative adverse respiratory events in children with upper respiratory tract infections. Anesthesiology 95:299-306
5. Bordet A, Allaouchiche D, Lansiaux S et al (2002) Risk factors for airway complications during general anaesthesia in pediatric patients. Pediatr Anesth 12:762-769
6. Schreiner MS, O'Hara L, Markakis DS et al (1996) Do children who experience laryngospasm have an increased risk of upper respiratory tract infection? Anesthesiology 85:475-480
7. Parnis S, Barker DS, van der Walt JH (2001) Clinical predictors of anaesthetic complications in children with respiratory tract infections. Pediatr Anesth 11:29-40
8. Cohen MM, Cameron CB (1991) Should you cancel the operation when a child has an upper respiratory tract infection? Anesth Analg 72:282-288
9. Jones AG (1993) Anaesthetic death of a child with a cold (letter). Anaesthesia 48:642
10. Konazerwski WH et al (1992) Anaesthetic death of a child with a cold. Anaesthesia 47:624

11. Critchley LA (1997) Yet another report of anaesthetic death due to unsuspected myocarditis. J Clin Anesth 19:676-677
12. Tabib A, Loire R, Miras A et al (2000) Unsuspected cardiac lesions associated with sudden unexpected perioperative death. Eur J Anaesthesiol 17:230-235
13. Van Ungern-Sternberg BS, Boda K, Chambers NA (2010) Risk assessment for respiratory complications in paediatric anaesthesia: a prospective cohort study. Lancet 376:773-783
14. Tait AR, Pandit UA, Voepel-Lewis T et al (1998) Use of laryngeal mask airway in children with upper respiratory tract infections: a comparison with endotracheal intubation. Anesth Analg 86:706-711
15. Asero R (2001) Multiple drug allergy syndrome: a distinct clinical entity. Curr Allergy Resp 1:18-22
16. Johansson SG, Bieber T, Dahl R et al (2004) Revised nomenclature for allergy for global use. J Allergy Clin Immunol 113:832-836
17. Dewachter P, Mouton-Faivre C, Emala CW (2009) Anaphylaxis and anesthesia: controversies and new insights. Anesthesiology 111:1141-1150
18. Kroigaard M, Garvey LH, Gillberg L et al (2007) Scandinavian Clinical Practice Guidelines on the diagnosis, management and follow-up of anaphylaxis during anaesthesia. Acta Anaesthesiol Scand 51:655-670
19. Dewachter P, Mouton-Faivre C (2008) What investigation after an anaphylactic reaction during anaesthesia? Curr Opin Anaesthesiol 21:363-368
20. Harper NJ, Dixon T, Dugue P et al (2009) Suspected anaphylactic reactions associated with anaesthesia. Anaesthesia 64:199-211
21. Clark AT, Skypala I, Leech SC et al (2010) British Society for Allergy and Clinical Immunology guidelines for the management of egg allergy. Clin Exp Allergy 40:1116-1129
22. De Leon-Casasola OA, Weiss A, Lema MJ (1992) Anaphylaxis due to propofol. Anesthesiology 77:384-386
23. Laxenaire MC, Mata-Bermejo E, Moneret-Vautrin DA, Gueant JL (1992) Life-threatening anaphylactoid reactions to propofol (Diprivan). Anesthesiology 77:275-280
24. Savage JH, Kaeding AJ, Matsui EC, Wood RA (2010) The natural history of soy allergy. J Allergy Clin Immunol 125:683-686
25. Lopata AL, O'Hehir RE, Lehrer SB (2010) Shellfish allergy. Clin Exp Allergy 40:850-858
26. Dewachter P, Tréchot P, Mouton-Faivre C (2005) 'Iodine allergy': point of view. Ann Fr Anesth Reanim 24:40-52
27. Guidelines for the Diagnosis and Management of Asthma, in National Asthma Education and Prevention Program Expert Panel (2007) The National Heart, Lung and Blood Institute
28. Woods BD, Sladen RN (2009) Peroperative considerations for the patient with asthmas and bronchospasm. Brit J Anaesth 103(BJA/PGA Supplement):i57-i65
29. Zachary CY, Evans R 3rd (1996) Perioperative management for childhood asthma. Ann Allergy Asthma Immunol 77:468-472
30. Qureshi F, Zaritsky A, Poirier MP (2001) Comparative efficacy of oral dexamethasone versus oral prednisone in acute pediatric asthma. J Pediatr 139:20-26
31. Pizov R, Brown RH, Weiss YS et al (1995) Wheezing during induction of general anesthesia in patients with and without asthma. A randomized, blinded trial. Anesthesiology 82:1111-1116
32. Scalfaro P, Sly PD, Sims C, Habre W (2001) Salbutamol prevents the increase of respiratory resistance caused by tracheal intubation during sevoflurane anesthesia in asthmatic children. Anesth Analg 93:898-902
33. Jenkins C, Costello J, Hodge L (2004) Systematic review of prevalence of aspirin induced asthma and its implications for clinical practice. BMJ 328:434

Anesthesia and Perioperative Safety in Children: Standards of Care and Quality Control

Paolo Murabito, Marinella Astuto, Giuliana Arena
and Antonino Gullo

9.1 Introduction

The perioperative care of infants and children requires specialized facilities and represents a challange for anesthesiologists. Many factors are involved in a positive outcome from surgery and anesthesia in children and both are down to strict organization and management and also to the experience of the clinical team [1].

Pediatric anesthesia presents a specific set of problems, as the age of the patients can vary widely (from premature neonates and infants to children and adolescents), each group having a specific anatomy, physiology, metabolism, and pathology; this makes pediatric anesthesia a highly specialized area within the wider disciplines of anesthesia and intensive care.

It has long been known that experienced surgical and anesthesia staff decrease mortality and morbidity in young patients considerably. Mortality associated with anesthesia has drammatically decreased from 6 per 10,000 of the population in the period 1947–1956 to 0.36 per 10,000 of the population in 2000 [2,3].

The reasons for this improvement can be ascribed to a new patient approach, the introduction of new drugs with better safety profiles, new and advanced technologies in patient monitoring and management, the adherence to approved standards of care and quality of care criteria and, furthermore, to a new training and educational system for health-care providers characterized by specific training in pediatric anesthesia and critical care.

P. Murabito (✉)
Department of Anaesthesia and Intensive Care
University Hospital Policlinico–Vittorio Emanuele
Catania, Italy
e-mail: paolomurabito@tiscali.it

M. Astuto (ed.) *Pediatric Anesthesia, Intensive Care and Pain: Standardization in Clinical Practice*. Anesthesia, Intensive Care and Pain in Neonates and Children
DOI: 10.1007/978-88-470-2685-8_9, © Springer-Verlag Italia 2013

9.2   Safety in Pediatric Anesthesia

Epidemiological data regarding anesthesia-related mortality and morbidity in pediatric patients are scarce. An interesting paper published in 2001 by Tay and colleagues [4] presented data regarding the spectrum of perioperative incidents seen in Singapore during 10,000 anesthesiological procedures in the period between 1997 and 1999.

The authors performed an audit for every case that required the presence of an anesthesiologist. On one side of the audit form, the attending anesthesiologist wrote a narrative description of the incident. The authors reported 297 incidents in 278 patients with the higher percentage of critical events in infants under 10 kg of weight. Most of the incidents happened during patient management and involved the respiratory system (approximately 78%), with laryngospasm being the most frequent cause.

This occurred most frequently during the immediate postinduction period compared with extubation or recovery time, and it was probably due to the stimulation produced by the transfer from the parent's lap onto the operating table [5].

Hemorrhage and hypotension were the most common incidents affecting the cardiovascular system. Only a few cases of dysrhythmias were reported: ventricular tachycardias, frequent ventricular ectopics, type II atrioventricular block, and bradycardia.

In contrast, Cohen and colleagues reported that dysrhythmias were the most frequent cardiovascular problem in children undergoing surgical procedures and anesthesia [6]. Organ impairment is not the only anesthesia-related incident. Other can be ascribed to the following elements.

9.2.1   Pharmacological Events
- Allergic reactions (antibiotics, local anesthetics, nonsteroidal anti-inflammatory drugs).
- Blood transfusion reaction.
- Syringe mislabeling.
- Incorrect administration [7].
- Drug toxicity [8,9].

Vigilance, by monitoring the depth of anesthesia to prevent an overdose, careful drug labeling, strict compliance with guidelines and recommendantions with regard to drug management and storage, all contribute to a significant reduction of anesthesia-related mortality.

9.2.2   Equipment Problems
- Disconnection of the breathing circuit.
- Occlusion of the breathing circuit.
- Anesthesia equipment malfunction.

9.2.3   Technique Difficulties
General anesthesia with regional techniques are always combined to guarantee a good intra- and postoperative pain control. Despite the high number of regional procedures performed, incidents are quite rare [4].

It is evident from the literature that the prevention of anesthesia-related incidents calls for many steps to be taken during the perioperative time. Before surgery patients should be carefully assessed and, if necessary, stabilized (blood pressure, heart rate, hydro-electrolyte and acid-base balance). All equipment and drugs should be strictly checked. The maintenance of anesthesia always requires the presence of the physician, and continous vigilance and patient monitoring as described in the guidelines.

Adherence to basic monitoring standards is essential to prevent errors, even if anesthesia is performed by an experienced and conscientious anesthesiologist. The necessary support and the implementation of national and local quality programs aimed at detecting critical situations or errors that may compromise patient safety, and strategies and protocols aimed at preventing and controlling recurrent errors, are essential to reduce anesthesia-induced mortality and morbidity [10].

9.3 Training and Education

Many countries have developed guidelines about pediatric health care, even though currently there are no agreed standards for the European Community as a whole [11–13].

Nevertheless, the Federation of European Associations of Paediatric Anaesthesia (FEAPA; now the European Society for Paediatric Anaesthesiology, distributed practical recommendations with the purpose of creating desirable standards for pediatric anesthesia services in Europe.

With regard to education in pediatric anesthesia, anesthesiologists must have specific training in the management of the pediatric patient and sufficient ongoing training to keep these skills up to date.

It is essential to bear in mind that all training should be competency-based with continous assessment and supervision. The number of procedures to be undertaken by a physician in training should only be taken as a guide and not as a legal requirement, even if it should be preferable to closely follow the FEAPA recommendations. The recommendations are subdivided into different categories according to the different career goals of each trainee [14].

9.3.1 All Trainees in Anesthesia (Regardless of Their Future Career)

A minimum of 3 months of continuous training provided in a specialist pediatric center in a University hospital, a large Children's Hospital or a District (nonspecialist) Hospital with a large pediatric department, or a combination thereof, that have all the facilities required for the management of children, is suggested. It is not only important to perform a sufficient number of procedures, but also for those procedures to involve a mixed-age group of patients:

- 10 infants less than 1 year of age (minimum two neonates).
- 20 children aged 1–3 years old.
- 60 children aged 3–10 years old.

At the end of the training period, all specialists in anesthesia and intensive care should be able to safely perform anesthesia procedures for common surgery in children over 3 years old and also to keep up to date with pediatric resuscitation and the stabilization of infants and children prior to transfer to a specialized center.

9.3.2 Trainees Interested in Pediatric Anesthesia

A further training module of at least 6 months continuous training is recommended. These specialists may work in units or hospitals in which they would be expected to undertake a minimum of half a day pediatric anesthesia per week (less than 50% of their working time) in pediatric activities. They should keep up to date with specific pediatric issues and they should periodically attend a specialized surgical center to maintain or improve their knowledge and expertise.

9.3.3 Trainees Who Want to Specialize in Pediatric Anesthesia

A further module of continuous training lasting for a minimum of 1 year and taking place in a specialized center is recommended. The surgical case mix should be extensive and should include emergency cases. Moreover, trainees are required to spend either 1 or 2 months in a pediatric intensive care unit, though not considering this as full training in this area as many countries require an additional period of training of up to 2 years.

Specialists in pediatric anesthesia are those physicians who spend at least 50% of their working time involved in the care of infants and children and who are qualified in the management of pediatric anesthesia, in resuscitation and emergency care, in the treatment of pain, and in the early stabilization of children requiring intensive care.

At the end of all formative steps, trainees will be expected to have attained knowledge of:

- The anatomical, physiological, and pharmacological differences between children and adults.
- The principles of resuscitation, and emergency and intensive care for children of all ages.
- The principles of safety and quality of pediatric care (e.g., transporting infants from a hospital to a specialized center).
- Technical skills (e.g., airway management, regional anesthesia, and analgesia).
- Medico-legal issues specific to pediatric practice (e.g., informed consent and clinical research).

These recommendations underline the importance of having a specialized clinical team and a pediatric intensive care bed available when necessary. Only in this way can services be delivered safely and promptly so as to handle emergencies effectively.

Agreement with these recommendations is not fully widespread in Italy. In 2006, Astuto and colleagues started to conduct a first survey to evaluate if the guidelines distributed by FEAPA had been adopted by the Italian postgraduate schools of anesthesia and intensive care or whether other training was being carried out. All the

Table 9.1 Initial survey carried out to evaluate the adoption of the FEAPA guidelines by Italian postgraduate schools of anesthesia and intensive care

Questionnaire
1. Does the school provide peditric training? If yes: what is the duration?
2. Are there a minimum number of procedures to perform during the training period?
3. Does the trainee have a test at the end of the training period?
4. Does your department have a team of anesthetists dedicated to pediatrics?

directors of the 37 Italian schools of anesthesia and intensive care were contacted and informed about the survey. A questionnaire, containing four simple questions (see Table 9.1), was distributed and the answers were collated in an electronic database and processed to obtain relevant information [15].

From the analysis of the completed questionnaires, it appeared that a minimum training in pediatric anesthesia is mandatory in the majority (92%) of the schools of anesthesia which took part in the survey. In 60% of the schools, training lasted for 3 months.

With regard to the minimum number of procedures provided for trainees by the FEAPA recommendations, including a large case mix and patients from all age groups, the results showed that only few institutions (29%) involved in a postgraduate educational program comply with these requirements.

Moreover, even though trainees should be formally evaluated both during and at the end of their pediatric training, the survey revealed that although Italian residents undergo formal assessment of their knowledge of and practice in pediatric anesthesia, the timing and form of such evaluation is not always standardized.

Currently, training in pediatric anesthesia is not a prerequisite for the anesthesia board examination in Italy, although those teaching hospitals that allow trainees to attend specific training have a dedicated group of pediatric anesthesiologists as supervisors for residents.

9.4   International Perspective

Other experiences worldwide have demonstrated that good training programs in pediatric anesthesia and intensive care were developed over 5 years ago and are now well established [13]. Comparing the results from Italian surveys with international educational systems, it is possible to state that resident training differs across the five continents.

In 2007, in a set of six surveys, Dent and colleagues reported on Australasian physician training in the emergency department involving pediatric patients [16–18]. One year later, the Australian and New Zealand College of Anaesthetists (ANZCA) approved a training sequence encompassing:
1. An initial 2-year prevocational medical education training period.

2. A 5-year period of ANZCA-approved training, during which period Fellows have to perform a minimum 50 half-day sessions of clinical activity, including anesthesia procedures in different surgical subspecialties (i.e., general surgery, neurosurgery, otolaryngology) and clinical management of important childhood conditions both in preoperative assessment and in emergency care (i.e., respiratory infections, prematurity and its complications, neonatal emergencies, congenital cardiac disease, facial anomalies affecting the airway) [19].

In Japan, training in pediatric anesthesia was evaluated by Shimada and colleagues, who reported that only a very low percentage of interviewees practiced pediatric anesthesia daily, while many did not practice it at all. These poor results are likely due to the fact that almost all anesthesia schools did not provide specific pediatric training, even if it was considered mandatory by the Japanese Society of Anesthesiologists [20].

Few studies on pediatric anesthesia have been published for the African continent. Some surveys report that only a few anesthesiologists were able to provide safe pediatric anesthesia [21] and there are no guidelines for anesthesia training.

In Chile, South America, thanks to the help of the World Federation of Societies of Anaesthesiologists, training in pediatric anesthesia is well established and consists of a training period lasting from 6 months to 1 year [22].

In North America, the situation changed in 1975 when Smith [23] described in his survey the development of pediatric anesthesia in the USA, indicating its importance. He also described an approved third-year residency offered by seven pediatric centers, which represented the first example of an experimental standardization in pediatric anesthesia training [23].

9.5 Clinical Setting

Pediatric patients are not small adults and so they need not only specialized medical staff but also a fit and suitable environment with all the appropriate facilities provided for them. The presence of parents is essential during the various clinical steps, including special areas like intensive care units or operating theaters [24].

Parents should be involved in all the aspects of the decision-making process and, for this reason, good and clear communication is fundamental for quality of care. Communication also involves the children, according to their age and comprehension ability. In the right circumstances, the young patients' consent should also be obtained.

Overnight accommodation should be available for parents whose children require admission to hospital, particularly if in critical situations.

Even technologies have to be specifically tailored to pediatric patients: warming devices should be available in the operating theater; the anesthesia equipment should provide mechanical pulmonary ventilation for children of all ages and weight; age-adjusted equipment and disposable items should be available for general and regional anesthesia.

9.6   Conclusions

Pediatric anesthesia should undoubtedly be viewed as a subspecialty addressing the entire pediatric population (from pre-term neonates to teenagers), which requires specific anatomical, pathophysiological, pharmacological, and anesthesiological knowledge. To prevent incidents and to guarantee optimal quality of care, many European countries have developed national guidelines to help health-care providers to work according to best practice principles.

Neverthless, there are many differences among national health systems; for this reason, FEAPA attempted to summarize all the requirements needed to foster an optimal pediatric environment in a unique document, which contains the main recommendations with regard to organization, safety, training and education, and clinical services and facilities.

However, strict adherence to all of these recommendations and guidelines is needed to reach the ultimate goal of "best practice" and thereby maximun safety for all our children.

References

1. Lunn JN, Devlin HB, Hoile RW, Campling EA (1993) Editorial II – the National Confidential Enquiry into Perioperative Deaths. Br J Anaesth 70(3):382
2. Short TG, O'Regan A, Jayasuriya JP (1996) Improvements in anaesthetic care resulting from a critical incident reporting programme. Anaesthesia 51(7):615-621
3. Morray JP, Geiduschek JM, Ramamoorthy C (2000) Anesthesia-related cardiac arrest in children: initial findings of the Pediatric Perioperative Cardiac Arrest (POCA) Registry. Anesthesiology 93(1):6-14
4. Tay CL, Tan GM, Ng SB (2001) Critical incidents in paediatric anaesthesia: an audit of 10 000 anaesthetics in Singapore. Paediatr Anaesth 11(6):711-718
5. Van der Walt JH, Sweeney DB, Runciman WB, Webb RK (1993) The Australian Incident Monitoring Study. Paediatric incidents in anaesthesia: an analysis of 2000 incident reports. Anaesth Intensive Care 21(5):655-658
6. Cohen MM, Cameron CB, Duncan PG (1990) Pediatric anesthesia morbidity and mortality in the perioperative period. Anesth Analg 70(2):160-167
7. Morray JP, Geiduschek JM, Caplan RA et al (1993) A comparison of pediatric and adult anesthesia closed malpractice claims. Anesthesiology 78(3):461-467
8. Holzman RS, van der Velde ME, Kaus SJ et al (1996) Sevoflurane depresses myocardial contractility less than halothane during induction of anesthesia in children. Anesthesiology 85(6):1260-1267
9. Gall O, Annequin D, Benoit G et al (2001) Adverse events of premixed nitrous oxide and oxygen for procedural sedation in children. Lancet 358(9292):1514-1515
10. Campling EA, Devlin HB, Lunn JN (1990) The report of the National Confidential Enquiry into Perioperative Deaths 1989. London: Disc to Print Ltd
11. Report of a Working Group (2001) Guidance on the provision of paediatric anaesthetic service. Thr Royal College Anaesthetists Bulletin 8:355-359
12. Melarkode K, Abdelaal A, Bass S (2009) Training in pediatric anesthesia for registrars – UK National survey. Paediatr Anaesth 19(9):872-878

13. Hansen TG (2009) Specialist training in pediatric anesthesia – the Scandinavian approach. Paediatr Anaesth. 19(5):428-433
14. The Federation of European Associations of Paediatric Anaesthesia (2004) Recommendations for Paediatric Anaesthesia Services. Minerva Anestesiologica 70(11):XXIX-XXXII
15. Astuto M, Lauretta D, Minardi C (2008) Does the Italiana pediatric anesthesia training program adequately prepare resident for future clinical practice? What should be done? Paediatr Anaesth 18(2):172-175
16. Dent AW, Asadpour A, Weiland TJ et al (2008) Australasian emergency physicians: a learning and educational needs analysis. Part one: background and methodology. Profile of FACEM. Emerg Med Australas 20(1):51-57
17. Paltridge D, Dent AW, Weiland TJ (2008) Australasian emergency physicians: a learning and educational needs analysis. Part two: confidence of FACEM for tasks and skills. Emerg Med Australas 20(1):58-65
18. Dent AW, Weiland TJ, Paltridge D (2008) Australasian emergency physicians: a learning and educational needs analysis. Part Four: CPD topics desired by emergency physicians. Emerg Med Australas 20(3):260-266
19. http://www.anzca.edu.au/trainees/atp/curriculum/module-8/overview
20. Shimada Y, Nishiwaki K, Sato K (2006) Pediatric anesthesia practice and training in Japan: a survey. Paediatr Anaesth 16(5):543-547
21. Hodges SC, Mijumbi C, Okello M et al (2007) Anaesthesia services in developing countries: defining the problems. Anaesthesia 62(1):4-11
22. Cavallieri S, Canepa P, Campos M (2009) Evolution of the WFSA education program in Chile. Paediatr Anaesth 19(1):33-34
23. Smith RM (1975) The pediatric anesthetist, 1950-1975. Anesthesiology 43(2):144-155
24. Giannini A (2007) Open intensive care units: the case in favour. Minerva Anestesiol 73(5):299-305. Epub 2006 Nov 20

Current Trends in Pediatric Regional Anesthesia

10

Noemi Vicchio, Valeria Mossetti and Giorgio Ivani

10.1 Review of Current Trends in Pediatric Regional Anesthesia

The pediatric anesthesiologist copes with respiratory depression on a daily basis because the surgical pediatric patient is always a patient under general anesthesia. Avoiding the major respiratory depressant drugs and reassuring parents using an alternative approach is mandatory from an ethical viewpoint. In our center, the pediatric patient undergoing plastic, thoracic, abdominal, urological, and orthopedic surgery does so under locoregional anesthesia (LRA) whenever possible.

Generally, LRA allows a safer anesthesia and postoperative period, with earlier tracheal extubation, gastrointestinal function recovery, and discharge from the intensive care unit and from hospital [1]. In interventions with moderate-to-severe pain, a single injection is followed by the placement of a catheter for continuous peripheral or central nerve block. The orthopedic patient in particular benefits from the continuous infusion of local anesthetic, as this increases the effectiveness of motor physiotherapy.

LRA involves several not uncommon risks that should be taken into account, particularly by the pediatric anesthesiologist. These are: the puncture of critical structures; toxic levels of the anesthetic; and intravascular injection of local anesthetic.

Child anatomy varies widely, depending on the stage of bone growth, and the thickness and hydration of the subcutaneous tissue. The likelihood of damaging the surrounding structures and of accidental intravascular injection increase when blind techniques are used. The execution of a nerve block using ultrasound guidance has been shown to be safer than traditional landmark techniques [2–5]; indeed, it allows the visualization of variations in anatomical relationships while avoiding the puncturing of important structures, such as the pleura in the case of a supraclavicular or infraclavicular brachial block, and vessel puncture of a

G. Ivani (✉)
Division of Pediatric Anesthesiology and Intensive Care
Regina Margherita Children's Hospital, Turin, Italy
e-mail: gioivani@libero.it

M. Astuto (ed.) *Pediatric Anesthesia, Intensive Care and Pain: Standardization in Clinical Practice*. Anesthesia, Intensive Care and Pain in Neonates and Children
DOI: 10.1007/978-88-470-2685-8_10, © Springer-Verlag Italia 2013

minor artery, such as the transverse cervical artery when a supraclavicular brachial block is used.

Children under 1 year of age are especially susceptible to the neurological and cardiac toxicity of local anesthetics, which in particular cause a reduced metabolism and hepatic blood flow. In addition, low levels of alpha-1-acid glycoprotein result in higher levels of pharmacologically active, unbound drug. It is then important to reduce the amount of local anesthetic being administered, and inject it slowly and with precise movements under direct visualization of the needle's tip. Latzke and colleagues demonstrated that the effective dose, 99% response volume of local anesthetic for sciatic nerve block was 0.10 mL/mm² of the cross-sectional nerve area [6].

Furthermore, studies have shown that ultrasound-guided nerve blocks lead to a reduction of 30–50% of the quantity of local anesthetic used to block, and therefore nerve blocks can be achieved with significantly smaller volumes of local anesthetics. Multiple nerve blocks can then be applied with the highest safety profile [2].

When executing a nerve block, general anesthesia can hide the early symptoms of systemic anesthetic toxicity. The poor sensitivity of both blood aspiration and test dose in anesthetized children increase the risk of unknown intravascular injection [7]. Ultrasound-guided techniques increase safety via direct visualization of the spread of local anesthetic around the blocked nerve or plexus. Independently of ultrasound guidance, to perform a safe block, it is essential to have continuous electrocardiographic and blood pressure monitoring, since the first signs of systemic toxicity are cardiac manifestations, in particular T-wave amplitude or ST segment changes; maintaining spontaneous ventilation is needed to detect the possible cessation of the respiratory drive [7]. Furthermore, all drugs and equipment necessary for the immediate management of possible complications must be available, the earliest of these to be used being lipid infusion [8].

In terms of the quality of intra- and postoperative analgesia, the execution of a block using ultrasound guidance has been shown to be much more effective than traditional techniques in terms of the quality of intra- and postoperative analgesia.

For upper extremity blocks, ultrasound-guided practice has been shown to cause a reduction in pneumothorax and inadvertent intravascular injection in children, albeit with some limitations. Bernards and colleagues recommended against performing interscalene blocks in anesthetized or heavily sedated adults or pediatric patients, because of the high risk of spinal cord injury as documented by case reports [9]; however, some authors disagree with these conclusions [10,11]. We cannot exclude that ultrasound guidance may eventually overcome this limitation, by verifying the site of the cervical vertebrae and with the direct visualization of local anesthetic diffusion; further studies are indeed needed. Furthermore, it is noteworthy that the interscalene brachial plexus block is associated with a 100% incidence of hemidiaphragmatic palsy and a low anesthetic volume appears to decrease the incidence only when performed at the level of nerve root C7 [12].

Supraclavicular and infraclavicular brachial plexus approaches are potentially dangerous blocks in children, whose anatomical structures are enclosed within small spaces; therefore ultrasound guidance permits their safer use in children [13,14]. Marhofer and colleagues recommend an infraclavicular approach instead of a supraclavicular one when there is a large dorsal scapular artery at the supraclavicular level or an infraclavicular approach with greater visibility [14]. The axillary brachial plexus block is a safe block also in traditional landmark techniques; however, it is difficult to block all the branches, including the muscolocutaneus nerve. Furthermore, the area is rich of vessel and there is a high risk of intravascular injection, even when every precautionary measure is taken. Ultrasound guidance helps in overcoming this aspect, while also allowing a dramatic reduction in the dose of local anesthetic used. It is worth bearing in mind that children have thin septa between the radial, median, and ulnar nerve, and thus a better anesthetic spread than in adult patients [15].

Before the diffusion of ultrasound guidance, an ilioinguinal/iliohypogastric block was associated with the use of high doses of local anesthetic and had a reputation for being difficult to perform, often with an unsatisfactory outcome. The blind technique with "fascial click," the technique most frequently performed by pediatric anesthesiologists, has a failure incidence of over 30%, which is not acceptable in modern anesthesia [16]. Weintraud argues that this high failure rate can be explained by the fact that the technique is based on studies conducted in adults. The high failure rate can then be explained by anatomical variations, a thicker subcutaneous layer, muscle development, and the incorrect distribution of local anesthetic [16,17].

The ilioinguinal/iliohypogastric block quickly became one of the most studied blocks with ultrasound guidance in pediatric patients, because of the obvious advantages. It has a 100% success rate when the targeted ilioinguinal/iliohypogastric nerves are visualized, reducing the volume of local anesthetic by six- to eightfold than that used in landmark techniques [18]. Such volume reduction means a reduction in the risk of toxicity but also in the risk of femoral palsy, an event possibly caused by excessive anesthetic spread that may delay ambulation and discharge [18].

Ultrasound-guided rectus sheath block, useful for midline surgical incisions and especially for umbilical hernia repair in children, is a simple and safe technique in which direct visualization avoids peritoneal, bowel, and mesenteric vessel puncture [3, 19]. This is valid also for the transversus abdominis plane (TAP) block, useful for abdominal surgical pain involving the T10–L1 nerves. In both cases, the identification of local anesthetic spread in the exact site increases pain control, both in quality and duration [20]. For rectus sheath block, the exact site through which local anesthetic has to spread is between the rectus abdominis muscle and the posterior aspect of the rectus sheath [3]. For TAP block, the local anesthetic has to spread between the transversus abdominis and the internal oblique abdominal muscle. In the study by Tran and colleagues [21], segmental nerves T10, T11, T12, and L1 were involved in the dye in 50%, 100%, 100%, and 93% of cases, respectively.

O'Sullivan and colleagues [22] reported that in penile block there was no significant difference between the ultrasound-guided technique versus the landmark technique, even if pain control in the pre-discharge stage was better with the former.

In order to increase safety, lower limb blocks should be chosen rather than central blocks, when possible. A large prospective French study showed that the incidence of complications related to pediatric LRA was very low (0.9/1000) and was related mainly to central blocks [23]. Moreover, unlike central blocks, peripheral blocks eliminate the risk of urinary retention, can be performed independently by coagulopathy, and limit the block to the surgical field.

In the case of lower limb blocks carried out using a blind injection, the block can appear incomplete [24] and ultrasound guidance, as shown by Oberndorfer and colleagues [5], increases the duration of sensory blockade when compared with nerve stimulator guidance, and prolongs the sensory blockade using smaller volumes of local anesthetic [5].

In pediatric patients and in particular in patients weighing less than 10–12 kg, visibility of the neuraxial structures is optimal when ultrasound is used. Being able to recognize the ligamentum flavum, dura madre, and epidural space is useful to confirm the correct positioning of the epidural catheter [25–27]. Another possible use of ultrasound guidance is to measure the angle and depth from the skin to the epidural space to guide the tip of the needle [28]. Rapp and colleagues [28] and Willschke and colleagues [29] positioned epidural catheters using real-time paramedian longitudinal probe position with reduction in bone contacts, faster catheter placement, and direct visualization of the local anesthetic spread. Limitations include the need for an assistant to handle the probe and the possible interference between the operator's hands, the needle, and the probe. Karmakar and colleagues used a real-time ultrasound-guided paramedian epidural access by means of a Tuohy needle/spring loaded syringe [30]. Perhaps this technique could also be piloted in children.

In caudal blocks, it is also important to detect the correct position of the needle to avoid intravascular or intrathecal injection, even if the risk is very low; therefore, ultrasound guidance has limited function in this context. However, in particular situations such as those involving obese patients or patients with a difficult anatomy, ultrasound guidance allows the identification of the sacral hiatus and the visualization of the cephalad spread [31].

Complications with ultrasound guidance are rare: the most frequent is the execution of an inadequate block; less frequent is nerve damage, which can be caused by a blunt needle of the correct size, but also by pressure injection of local anesthetic. A high injection pressure means that the needle is in an intraneural position, with high risk of severe and/or persistent neurological injury [32].

In addition to ultrasound guidance, known essential factors for reducing the risks and increasing the effectiveness of LRA are the levo enantiomer local anesthetics, ropivacaine and levobupivacaine, if possible combined with adjuvants. Levobupivacaine and ropivacaine compared with a racemic mixture have reduced cardiovascular and neurotoxicity. Additionally, a more selective sensory block tends to save the motor component [33–35]. The injection should be carried out slowly and after proof of aspiration, even if under ultrasound guidance. To increase safety, it can also be combined with adjuvants such as clonidine and ketamine to reduce the amount of local anesthetic to be administered and to extend the analgesic effect, with negligible side effects [36–45].

A balance between the efficacy of an anesthetic block and patient safety remains a major challenge for pediatric regional anesthesia. Ultrasound guidance is the main tool we have at our disposal and we need to disseminate the need for this fundamental technique.

References

1. Bösenberg A (2004) Pediatric regional anesthesia update. Paediatr Anaesth 14(5):398-402
2. Willschke H, Marhofer P, Bösenberg A et al (2005) Ultrasonography for ilioinguinal/ilio-hypogastric nerve blocks in children. British Journal of Anaesthesia 95:226-230
3. Willschke H, Bösenberg A, Marhofer P et al (2006) Ultrasonography-guided rectus sheath block in paediatric anaesthesia – a new approach to an old technique. British Journal of Anaesthesia 97:244-249
4. Marhofer P, Sitzwohl C, Greher M, Kapral S (2004) Ultrasound guidance for infraclavicular brachial plexus anaesthesia in children. Anaesthesia 59:642-646
5. Oberndorfer U, Marhofer P, Bösenberg A et al (2007) Ultrasonographic guidance for sciatic and femoral nerve blocks in children. Br J Anaesth 98(6):797-801
6. Latzke D, Marhofer P, Zeitlinger M et al (2010) Minimal local anaesthetic volumes for sciatic nerve block: evaluation of ED 99 in volunteers. Br J Anaesth 104(2):239-244
7. Mossetti V, Ivani G (2012) Controversial issues in pediatric regional anesthesia. Paediatr Anaesth 22(1):109-114
8. Weinberg GL (2010) Treatment of local anesthetic systemic toxicity (LAST). Reg Anesth Pain Med 35:188-193
9. Bernards CM, Hadzic A, Suresh S, Neal JM (2008) Regional anesthesia in anesthetized or heavily sedated patients. Reg Anesth Pain Med 33(5):449-460
10. Bogdanov A, Loveland R (2005) Is there a place for interscalene block performed after induction of general anaesthesia? Eur J Anaesth, 22:107-110
11. Devera HV, Furukawa KT, Scavone JA et al (2009) Interscalene blocks in anesthetized pediatric patients. Reg Anesth Pain Med 34(6):603-604
12. Renes SH, Rettig HC, Gielen MJ et al (2009) Ultrasound-guided low-dose interscalene brachial plexus block reduces the incidence of hemidiaphragmatic paresis. Reg Anesth Pain Med 34(5):498-502
13. Yang CW, Cho CK, Kwon HU et al (2010) Ultrasound-guided supraclavicular brachial plexus block in pediatric patients – A report of four cases. Korean J Anesthesiol 59(Suppl):S90-S94
14. Marhofer P, Willschke H, Kettner SC (2012) Ultrasound-guided upper extremity blocks – tips and tricks to improve the clinical practice. Paediatr Anaesth 22(1):65-71
15. Willschke H, Marhofer P, Machata AM, Lönnqvist PA (2010) Current trends in paediatric regional anaesthesia. Anaesthesia 65(Suppl 1):S97-S104
16. Weintraud M, Marhofer P, Bösenberg A et al (2008) Ilioinguinal/iliohypogastric blocks in children: where do we administer the local anesthetic without direct visualization? Anesthesia & Analgesia 106:89-93
17. Hong JY, Kim WO, Koo BN et al (2010) The relative position of ilioinguinal and iliohypogastric nerves in different age groups of pediatric patients. Acta Anaesthesiol Scand 54(5):566-570
18. Willschke H, Bösenberg A, Marhofer P et al (2006) Ultrasonographic-guided ilioinguinal/iliohypogastric nerve block in pediatric anesthesia: what is the optimal volume? Anesth Analg 102(6):1680-1684
19. Ferguson S, Thomas V, Lewis I (1996) The rectus sheath block in paediatric anaesthesia: new indications for an old technique? Paediatr Anaesth 6(6):463-466
20. Fredrickson M, Seal P, Houghton J (2008) Early experience with the transversus abdominis plane block in children. Paediatr Anaesth 18(9):891-892
21. Tran TM, Ivanusic JJ, Hebbard P, Barrington MJ (2009) Determination of spread of injectate after ultrasound-guided transversus abdominis plane block: a cadaveric study. Br J Anaesth 102(1):123-127
22. O'Sullivan MJ, Mislovic B, Alexander E (2011) Dorsal penile nerve block for male pediatric circumcision – randomized comparison of ultrasound – guided vs anatomical landmark technique. Paediatr Anaesth 21(12):1214-1218
23. Ecoffey C, Lacroix F, Giaufré E et al (2010)Association des Anesthésistes Réanimateurs Pédiatriques d'Expression Française (ADARPEF). Epidemiology and morbidity of regional

anesthesia in children: a follow-up one-year prospective survey of the French-Language Society of Paediatric Anaesthesiologists (ADARPEF). Paediatr Anaesth 20(12):1061-1069

24. Vas L (2005) Continuous sciatic block for leg and foot surgery in 160 children. Paediatr Anaesth 15(11):971-978

25. Marhofer P, Bösenberg A, Sitzwohl C et al (2005) Pilot study of neuraxial imaging by ultrasound in infants and children. Paediatr Anaesth 15(8):671-676

26. Kil HK, Cho JE, Kim WO et al (2007) Prepuncture ultrasound-measured distance: an accurate reflection of epidural depth in infants and small children. Reg Anesth Pain Med 32(2):102-106

27. Chawathe MS, Jones RM, Gildersleve CD et al (2003) Detection of epidural catheters with ultrasound in children. Paediatr Anaesth 13(8):681-684

28. Rapp HJ, Folger A, Grau T (2005)Ultrasound-guided epidural catheter insertion in children. Anesth Analg 101(2):333-339

29. Willschke H, Marhofer P, Bösenberg A et al (2006) Epidural catheter placement in children: comparing a novel approach using ultrasound guidance and a standard loss-of-resistance technique. Br J Anaesth 97(2):200-207

30. Karmakar MK, Li X, Ho AM et al (2009) Real-time ultrasound-guided paramedian epidural access: evaluation of a novel in-plane technique. Br J Anaesth 102(6):845-854

31. Schwartz D, Raghunathan K, Dunn S, Connelly NR (2008) Ultrasonography and pediatric caudals. Anesth Analg 106(1):97-99

32. Hadzic A, Dilberovic F, Shah S et al (2004)Combination of intraneural injection and high injection pressure leads to fascicular injury and neurologic deficits in dogs. Reg Anesth Pain Med 29(5):417-423

33. Ecoffey C (2005) Local anesthetics in pediatric anesthesia: an update. Minerva Anestesiol 71(6):357-360

34. Ivani G, De Negri P, Lonnqvist PA (2005) Caudal anesthesia for minor pediatric surgery: a prospective randomized comparison of ropivacaine 0.2% vs levobupivacaine 0.2%. Paediatr Anaesth 15(6):491-494

35. De Negri P, Ivani G, Tirri T (2005) New local anesthetics for pediatric anesthesia. Curr Opin Anaesthesiol 18(3):289-292

36. Dahmani S, Michelet D, Abback PS et al (2011) Ketamine for perioperative pain management in children: a meta-analysis of published studies. Paediatr Anaesth 21(6):636-652

37. De Negri P, Ivani G, Visconti C, De Vivo P (2001) How to prolong postoperative analgesia after caudal anaesthesia with ropivacaine in children: S-ketamine versus clonidine. Paediatr Anaesth 11(6):679-683

38. Locatelli BG, Frawley G, Spotti A et al (2008) Analgesic effectiveness of caudal levobupivacaine and ketamine. Br J Anaesth 100(5):701-706

39. Kumar P, Rudra A, Pan AK, Acharya A (2005) Caudal additives in pediatrics: a comparison among midazolam, ketamine, and neostigmine coadministered with bupivacaine. Anesth Analg 101(1):69-73

40. Passariello M, Almenrader N, Canneti A et al (2004) Caudal analgesia in children: S(+)-ketamine vs S(+)-ketamine plus clonidine. Paediatr Anaesth. 14(10):851-855

41. Cucchiaro G, Ganesh A (2007) The effects of clonidine on postoperative analgesia after peripheral nerve blockade in children. Anesth Analg 104(3):532-537

42. Nishina K, Mikawa K (2002) Clonidine in paediatric anesthesia. Curr Opin Anaesthesiol 15(3):309-316

43. Ivani G, De Negri P, Conio A et al (2000) Ropivacaine-clonidine combination for caudal blockade in children. Acta Anaesthesiol Scand 44(4):446-449

44. De Negri P, Ivani G, Visconti C et al (2001) The dose-response relationship for clonidine added to a postoperative continuous epidural infusion of ropivacaine in children. Anesth Analg 93(1):71-76

45. Bergendahl GHT, Lonnqvist PA, De Negri P et al (2002) Increased postoperative arterial blood pressure stability with continuous epidural infusion of clonidine in children. Anesth Analg 95(4):1121-1122

Locoregional Anesthesia in Children

11

Adrian T. Bosenberg

11.1 Introduction

Worldwide pediatric regional anesthesia continues to evolve. In some countries, regional anesthesia forms part of the "anesthetic culture" and it is almost an anticipated to provide analgesia for children after surgery. In some institutions, the use of regional anesthesia in children remains limited because of the perception that the advantages of regional anesthesia over opiate analgesia [1,2] are not worth the potential risks. Although different, the incidence of risk associated with regional anesthesia is remarkably similar to opiate analgesia, i.e., approximately 1 per 1,000 of the population, based on recent multicenter surveys [3,4].

In choosing regional anesthesia, the risks and benefits of any technique must be weighed against the risks and benefits of other forms of analgesia. Many factors influence the choice of technique and include: the age and general condition of the patient; the severity and site of the pain; informed consent; the skill of the provider; and whether any contraindication to regional anesthesia exists. In making the choice, the anesthesiologist should also take into account the availability of equipment, and the facilities and level of both monitoring and nursing care available [2]. In general terms, a peripheral nerve block is considered safer than a neuraxial block.

11.2 Benefits

Untreated pain has several deleterious effects, whereas effective pain relief may play an important role in surgical outcome. Regional anesthesia is almost universally employed to provide analgesia, but it may also be used for its autonomic and

A.T. Bosenberg (✉)
Department Anesthesiology and Pain Management
Faculty of Health Sciences, University of Washington, Seattle Children's Hospital
Seattle, USA
e-mail: adrian.bosenberg@seattlechildrens.org

M. Astuto (ed.) *Pediatric Anesthesia, Intensive Care and Pain: Standardization in Clinical Practice.* Anesthesia, Intensive Care and Pain in Neonates and Children
DOI: 10.1007/978-88-470-2685-8_11, © Springer-Verlag Italia 2013

motor effects in special circumstances. Surgical stress, if untreated, produces a spectrum of autonomic, hormonal, metabolic, immunological-inflammatory, and neurobehavioral consequences. Regional anesthesia is most effective in blunting this response.

It is difficult to show clear, "evidence-based" benefits of regional anesthesia over other forms of analgesia [1,3–6]. With respect to the pyramid of evidence, apart from many single institution case series, retrospective reviews, and anecdotal reports, there are few prospective randomized control studies comparing regional with general anesthesia or systemic analgesics in children [2]. Those that have been performed are often underpowered, have different and varying end points, and are usually from single institutions. Another confounding factor is that more surgery is being done laparoscopically or thoracoscopically, requiring a different analgesic technique than that used for open laparotomy or thoracotomy [7,8].

Bearing this in mind, there is some evidence to suggest that the benefits of regional anesthesia in children include hemodynamic stability and a reduction in minimum alveolar concentration; less need for muscle relaxants; absence of respiratory depression with some evidence of respiratory stimulation; less need for postoperative ventilatory support after major surgery (particularly thoracotomy); earlier return of gut function and subsequent feeding; enhanced suppression of the metabolic stress response; and less immunodepression, in addition to the economic benefits of a shorter intensive care unit and hospital stay [1,2].

11.3 Education

Success in regional blockade involves placing "the right dose of the right drug in the right place." To achieve this goal, individual practitioners require sufficient education and training to acquire the confidence to practice independently.

Anatomy remains the foundation on which regional anesthesia is built. Pediatric anatomy is somewhat different from that of adults and evolves as the child grows. On the positive side, most nerves are superficial and therefore can be better defined with high-frequency ultrasound and, for those practitioners who are restricted to nerve stimulation, nerve mapping is also easier when nerves are superficial. While ultrasound guidance has virtually become the standard of care in the developed world, nerve stimulation still has its place. After all, not so long ago, peripheral nerve stimulators were regarded a major advance, both as a teaching aid and as a means to improve the success rate of peripheral nerve blocks.

An understanding of anatomy, pattern recognition, hand–eye coordination, and optimal needle visualization remain the hallmarks of safe ultrasound-guided practice. Performing an ultrasound-guided block depends primarily on the operator's ability to locate the nerve, to follow and advance the needle tip toward the target nerve, and to a lesser extent on the ultrasound equipment and needle available. As the use of ultrasound expands, the best method of teaching is worth considering.

To date, training in ultrasound-guided nerve blocks has not been standardized [9]. Guidelines have been suggested, but most are aimed at the practice for adults [9–14]. The role of phantoms in teaching ultrasound-guided regional anesthesia has recently been reviewed [13]. Simulation of needle control on phantoms is popular and cost-effective without risk to patients. However, they are not ideal since a lack of background echogenicity greatly enhances needle visibility that does not resemble the clinical situation [13]. Animal models and fresh frozen cadavers are expensive, but are more realistic [13]. However, the use of pediatric cadavers is not an option. The plethora of workshops that have become available are mainly adult-orientated and invariably offer the basics only. Time allocated for individual hands-on experience is invariably limited and seldom involves needle insertion into live models.

The ideal is experience gained clinically under expert guidance. These opportunities remain limited to a minority of institutions worldwide. The suggested need for ultrasound certification should not, in the author's opinion, become a requirement unless there is real evidence that ultrasound-guided blocks are truly safer than nerve stimulator techniques.

11.4 Quality Improvement

In this era of evidence-based medicine, coupled with clinical practice that is becoming increasingly risk-averse [2], quality improvement and the safety of regional anesthesia should be an important focus both now and in the future. Should regional anesthesia remain the domain of enthusiasts or should it be more widely adopted and become a standard of practice? This remains a topic for debate. Regional anesthesia clearly has wide-ranging benefits [1], but requires technical expertise that is still not universally taught [9–12].

A review of four large prospective multicenter surveys, two from the Association Des Anesthésistes Réanimateurs Pédiatriques D'Expression Française (ADARPEF; the French-Language Societies of Pediatric Anesthesiologists) representative of two different eras [15,16], one from the UK [3], and more recently from the Pediatric Regional Anesthesia Network (PRAN) in the USA [8,17], show a remarkable similar incidence of non-life-threatening complications. The initial ADARPEF study, published in 1996, represented regional anesthesia prior to the advent of ultrasound guidance [15]. The most recent ADARPEF study, using the same methodology and comprising 31,132 regional blocks, reported the increased use of peripheral nerve blocks and continuous nerve blocks [16]. The PRAN survey, now with more than 40,000 blocks in its database, has shown a similar trend that is probably indicative of the increased use of laparoscopic surgery or is prompted by fewer complications associated with peripheral nerve blocks noted in earlier surveys [15,16].

What has not been resolved, despite the many advantages of ultrasound, is whether ultrasound-guided blocks are safer than those performed using a nerve stimulator.

Meta-analyses of early pediatric studies and studies in adults were inconclusive [18]. Ultrasound-guided nerve blocks are the fashionable expectation in our gadget-orientated society and have virtually become the standard of practice in affluent societies. But less affluent societies should not abandon nerve stimulation and forsake more important equipment, such as pulse oximetry [19], for the relatively small gain provided by ultrasound.

11.5 New Approaches

Recent reviews [20–23] and a special themed issue of *Pediatric Anesthesia* [20] have focused on the various aspects of regional anesthesia in infants and children. All, written by experienced practitioners and including manuscripts on neuraxial (epidural, caudal, spinal) and peripheral nerve blocks (upper and lower limb, truncal), and head and neck blocks, are valuable resources. Renewed interest in some peripheral nerve blocks recently described in children is the focus of this section.

11.5.1 Maxillary Nerve Blocks

Cleft palate surgery is not only painful but may also compromise the airway, particularly in those children with craniofacial syndromes. Opiate analgesia has the potential to further compromise the airway, whereas bilateral maxillary nerve block can provide analgesia without the risk of respiratory depression in these vulnerable patients. The approach to the maxillary nerve differs from that in adults since the facial configuration in infants undergoes changes with growth and development. Bilateral maxillary nerve block is thus performed using a suprazygomatic approach and is based on a computerized tomography study [24]. Despite the bony nature of the area, an ultrasound approach is also feasible [25]. The block is remarkably easy to perform with early indications of a low complication rate, and it seems to improve pain relief, decrease perioperative consumption of opioids, and favor early feeding resumption after cleft palate repair in infants [24].

11.5.2 Transversus Abdominis Plane Blocks

The transversus abdominis plane (TAP) block has also been described recently for pain management following abdominal surgery in infants and children [26]. The midaxillary line in-plane approach used in adults for the ultrasound-guided TAP block is not always feasible in small children because access to the space between the thoracic cage and the iliac crest is limited. An anterior–posterior in-plane approach–with probe almost vertical to the bed–is more user-friendly for infants and children.

The appropriate dosing guidelines and extent of spread of local anesthesia have been subject to debate and may explain the mixed success achieved with this block when used for upper and lower abdominal surgery. The extent of the spread using 0.2 mL/kg–the recommended pediatric guideline–has been questioned. The unpredictability of TAP blocks was demonstrated in a recent study, where the dermatomal spread was assessed in 35 blocks using 0.4 mL/kg [26]. The median level of blockade ranged from T10 to L1 in 75% of the children. Therefore, it has been argued that TAP blocks should be offered for lower abdominal surgery only [26]. In the author's opinion, TAP blocks are most useful for open appendectomy, colostomy closure, and inguinal and other lower abdominal surgery.

While technically challenging in a neonate because of their compliant abdominal wall, TAP blocks have been used as an alternative to neuraxial blocks or wound infiltration to provide analgesia for both major and minor neonatal surgery.

11.5.3 Lumbar Plexus Blocks

Lumbar plexus blocks are considered difficult blocks to perform in view of the potential risks involved [27, 28]. The femoral, obturator, and lateral femoral cutaneous nerves supplying the anterior aspect of the lower limb are more reliably blocked with a lumbar plexus block than a 3-in-1 nerve block. Several approaches to the lumbar plexus that rely on bony contact with the transverse process of L4 have been described in adults. In children, the transverse processes are not fully developed and using the transverse process as a guide places the needle too medial and increases the risk of puncturing a dural cuff on the spinal roots, or causing retrograde epidural spread to the opposite side.

Ultrasound guidance, while feasible, is limited to younger children because the definition obtained with linear probes from portable ultrasound units is inadequate for accurate placement if the lumbar plexus is deeper than 4–5 cm. Many advocate combining ultrasound with a nerve stimulator. An approach that the author has found useful is a modification of Winnie's approach. With the child in a lateral position, an insulated needle inserted perpendicular to the skin at the point where a line drawn from the posterior superior iliac spine, parallel to the spinous processes of the vertebrae, intersects the intercristal (Tuffier's) line, will advance through the posterior lumbar fascia, paraspinous muscles, anterior lumbar fascia, quadratus lumborum and onto the psoas muscle [27]. Passage through these fascial layers may be detected by distinct "pops" when using a short bevel needle. Quadriceps muscle twitches in the ipsilateral thigh are sought, confirming stimulation of the lumbar plexus. The depth from the skin to the lumbar plexus is approximately the same distance as the posterior superior iliac spine is to the intercristal line [27]. The depth of the needle is emphasized because of the complications associated with wayward needle advancement into the peritoneum or retroperitoneum that may result in renal hematoma, vascular puncture (retroperitoneal hematoma), or even bowel puncture.

11.6   Methods to Increase the Duration of Analgesia

11.6.1 Continuous Peripheral Nerve Blocks

Continuous peripheral nerve catheters have not been readily available for use in children until recently. Now, continuous postoperative pain management or pain therapy is feasible for older children and adolescents [29]. The main indications are for children undergoing procedures, or for conditions that are associated with significant or prolonged postoperative pain: to improve peripheral perfusion after microvascular surgery or in vasospastic disorders involving the limbs. In selected cases, patient-controlled analgesia is also feasible. Continuous infusions have also been used to provide analgesia to allow physical therapy in chronic regional pain syndromes. The blood levels of local anesthetic agents reached during continuous brachial plexus infusions are less than those reached during continuous epidural analgesia. Accurate placement can be confirmed with real-time ultrasound imaging or fluoroscopically.

For the lower extremity, the main indication has been the management of femur fracture or major trauma involving the lower limbs. Catheters have also been placed in the lumbar plexus or fascia iliaca compartment to provide unilateral analgesia of the hip or thigh. Fixation of the catheters for continuous use is considered easier on the lower extremity [30], particularly for lumbar plexus blocks [27].

Ideally, a commercially available kit should be used as they allow the use of a nerve stimulator to identify the nerve sheath prior to placement of the catheter. Several manufacturers now provide insulated Tuohy needles of "child-friendly" length through which an appropriately sized catheter can be passed. The role of stimulating versus nonstimulating catheters for continuous peripheral nerve blocks is the subject of ongoing research.

The dosage recommended for continuous infusions after an initial bolus dose are 0.1–0.2 mL/kg/h of either bupivacaine or levobupivacaine (0.125–0.25%) or ropivacaine (0.15–0.2%). The lower rates are generally used for upper extremity catheters and the higher rates for lower extremity nerve or plexus analgesia. The infusion rate may be adjusted as needed up to the maximum recommended infusion rates of 0.2 mg/kg/h for infants less than 6 months and 0.4 mg/kg/h in children older than 6 months. Elastomeric devices or disposable infusion pumps, that may be programmed to deliver local anesthetic based on a child's weight, are currently available and may offer an option for outpatient pediatric pain control in the future [29]. To date, the reported complications have been low but include catheter-induced infection, particularly in immunocompromised patients; hematoma formation; catheter breakage; or knot formation on removal.

11.6.2 Adjuvants

Adjuvants are drugs that increase the *efficacy or potency* of other drugs when given concurrently. Adjuvants, are used firstly to prolong the duration of analgesia after single-shot caudal blocks and secondly to improve the quality of the analgesia while allowing lower local anesthetic concentrations to be used, thereby reducing the unwanted side effects of local anesthetics, such as motor blockade and local anesthetic toxicity.

Single-shot caudals with bupivacaine, ropivacaine, or levobupivacaine are safe and effective but only provide analgesia for 4–6 h [31]. Since continuous infusions of local anesthetic agents have a relatively narrow margin of safety in young infants and children, a variety of agents have been used as adjuvants to prolong the analgesic efficacy of caudal, neuraxial, and even peripheral nerve blockade [32,33]. In choosing an adjuvant, the anesthesia provider must balance the benefits against the potential risks taking the age of the child and the impact of comorbidities into account, as well as the facilities available, in addition to whether the child is to be managed in hospital or at home.

Based on current evidence, it is difficult to reach a consensus on the most effective adjuvant. There is even less evidence when combinations are used. Most studies in children have used minor surgery (inguinal hernia repair, circumcision) under caudal block as the clinical research model. The heterogeneity of these studies, both in terms of the type and concentration of local anesthetic agent, as well as the dose of adjuvant used, are all confounding factors that make meta-analyses difficult [34,35]. The studies also vary in the nature of surgery, the premedication used, the method of pain assessment, and the age range of the children. Two surveys of members of the Association of Paediatric Anaesthetists of Great Britain and Ireland show an increase in the use of adjuvants to enhance the analgesia provided by a caudal block from 58% to almost 80% [36] over the past decade.

Although many other agents have been studied, the most effective agents in clinical practice are opiates (morphine, diamorphine), clonidine, and ketamine. Clonidine and ketamine have become increasingly popular, while opiates seem to be on the decline predominantly because of their unwanted side effects [36]. Ketamine, particularly racemic ketamine, despite its popularity in some countries, may suffer a similar fate as morphine in view of concerns related to neurotoxicity [35].

Clonidine, an alpha-2 adrenergic receptor agonist, has sedative, analgesic, and antihypertensive properties and is commercially available as a preservative-free preparation. There is good evidence that the major effect of clonidine is mediated at the spinal cord level [37]. Clonidine 1–2 µg/kg is effective and typically doubles the duration of the local anesthetic agent. Higher doses are associated with increasing sedation, bradycardia, hypotension, and a risk of apnea, particularly in neonates and infants. Clonidine (0.1 µg/kg/h) enhances the analgesia of dilute continuous epidural infusions of 0.1% bupivacaine or ropivacaine [34].

A meta-analysis of 20 randomized controlled trials (published between 1994 and 2010) including 993 patients (2–6 years old) undergoing urogenital or lower limb surgery showed a longer duration of postoperative analgesia in those receiving clonidine 0.1 µg/kg in addition to local anesthetic [mean duration (MD): 3.72 h; 95% confidence interval (CI): 2.61–4.84; $p < 0.00001$] with a lower risk of rescue analgesia [relative risk (RR): 0.72; 95% CI: 0.57–0.90; $p = 0.003$] than local anesthetic alone [34].

Clonidine seems to have a large margin of safety, based on three cases where 100 times the intended dose of caudal clonidine was administered to children 14 months–5 years without any untoward cardiorespiratory effects. All were somnolent for 24 h and made a full recovery. Several cases of respiratory depression and apnea have been reported in pre-term and term neonates, probably related to the immature respiratory control and central sedation. Clonidine is therefore not recommended for infants, particularly pre-term infants, less than 3 months of age in view of this risk of apnea.

Ketamine, a noncompetitive spinal N-Methyl-D-aspartate and mild mu-opiate receptor agonist, is most effective as an adjuvant for caudal block at doses of 0.25–1 mg/kg [35]. The same dose given intravenously has a much shorter duration of action, but given caudally ketamine can exceed clonidine. Higher doses increase the incidence of unwanted side effects (sedation, hallucinations, nystagmus, nausea, and vomiting) with little further improvement in analgesia.

In a similar quantitative review and meta-analysis of 13 randomized controlled trials (published between 1991 and 2008) that included 584 patients (2–12 years old) who underwent urogenital or lower limb surgery, ketamine 0.25–0.5 mg/kg combined with a single dose of local anesthetic (ropivacaine, bupivacaine) had a longer duration of analgesia (MD: 5.6 h; 95% CI: 5.45–5.76; $p < 0.00001$) with a lower RR of rescue analgesia (RR: 0.71; 95% CI: 0.44–1.15; $p = 0.16$) than local anesthetic alone, despite the heterogeneity of groups in the different studies [35].

The preservatives (benzethonium chloride, chlorbutanol) in the commercially available product have been implicated in the histopathological changes demonstrated in animal models but not in humans. This has raised concerns in some quarters. Despite numerous studies showing no ill effects, ketamine is no longer recommended as an adjuvant in Austria, Germany, and Switzerland. Preservative-free racemic ketamine and S(+)-ketamine are available in some countries. S(+)-ketamine has twice the analgesic potency of the racemate with fewer side effects.

Although both clonidine and ketamine increase the duration of analgesia, when used in combination S(+)-ketamine and clonidine can provide satisfactory analgesia for up to 20 h. To put this in perspective, it is worth considering that other regional techniques such as penile blocks, TAP blocks, and ilioinguinal blocks may offer longer or comparable duration of analgesia without the concerns outlined above.

It is difficult to advocate the use of other drugs containing potentially harmful preservatives or any drug that has not undergone proper safety evaluation. Agents such as midazolam, neostigmine, and to a lesser extent tramadol and buprenorphine, fall into this category. All produce limited increase in analgesia but are associated with an unacceptably high incidence of nausea and vomiting.

11.6.3 Peripheral Nerve Block Adjuvants

A variety of adjuvants have been used to supplement local anesthetics in peripheral nerve blocks with mixed results. A qualitative systematic review of 27 studies in adults where clonidine was used in peripheral nerve blocks proved inconclusive [38].

Until recently, there have been few studies in children. In a retrospective audit of 220 children (2–19 years old) at one institution who received clonidine in combination with bupivacaine or ropivacaine for a variety of blocks (brachial and lumbar plexus blocks, femoral, fascia iliaca, or sciatic nerve blocks), it was found that the sensory block was extended by a few hours but the incidence of motor block was increased compared to 215 children who had received plain bupivacaine or ropivacaine.

Clonidine did not prolong the duration of ilioinguinal blocks with 0.25% bupivacaine in 98 children between 1 and 12 years of age undergoing inguinal hernia surgery [39]. Clonidine did not improve the quality of analgesia but did prolong the duration of analgesia of an axillary block with 0.2% ropivacaine in 30 children aged from 1 to 6 years [39].

These findings are not surprising since there are no alpha-2-adrenergic receptors in peripheral nerves [40]. Based on animal studies, the mechanism of action is thought to be either by vasoconstriction or possibly via membrane hyperpolarization-activated cation currents [40].

11.7 Conclusions

Pediatric regional anesthesia continues to grow, particularly in the day surgery setting, for the many advantages outlined [2]. Patient safety should remain our focus when performing regional anesthesia. The choice of regional technique should be considered within the context of risk versus benefit based on the age of the child, the nature of the surgery, the facilities and equipment available, and the skill of the practitioner.

Technological advances in the future will improve the image quality of ultrasonography. The challenge in the future will be to determine which modality will be the most cost-effective to further broaden the horizons of pediatric regional anesthesia.

Regional anesthesia cannot move forward without the support of the whole surgical team. Education at all levels–surgeon, nurse, patient, family, as well as our anesthesiologist colleagues and trainees–is essential, particularly when continuous infusions are used. A successful block sells itself. The challenge for the future is to achieve success safely and to reduce the documented risk further.

References

1. Bosenberg A (2012) Benefits of regional anesthesia in children Paediatr Anaesth 22:10-18.
2. Bosenberg AT, Jöhr M, Wolf AR (2011) Pro con debate: the use of regional vs systemic analgesia for neonatal surgery. Paediatr Anaesth 21:1247-1258.
3. Llewellyn N, Moriarty A (2007)The national pediatric epidural audit. Paediatr Anaesth 17:520-533.

4. Morton NS, Errera A (2010) APA national audit of pediatric opioid infusions. Pediatr Anesth 20:119-125.
5. Polaner DM, Drescher J (2011) Pediatric regional anesthesia: what is the current safety record? Pediatr Anesth 21:737-742.
6. Willschke H, Marhofer P, Machata AM, Lönnqvist PA (2010) Current trends paediatric regional anaesthesia. Anaesthesia 65 Suppl 1:97-104.
7. Rochette A, Dadure C, Raux O et al (2007) A review of pediatric regional anesthesia practice during a 17-year period in a single institution. Pediatr Anesth 17:874-880.
8. Polaner DM, Martin LD; PRAN Investigators (2012) Quality assurance and improvement: the Pediatric Regional Anesthesia Network. Paediatr Anaesth 22:115-119.
9. Tsui BCH, Hui Yun Ip V (2011) Ultrasound beyond regional anesthesia Can J Anesth 58:499-503.
10. Regional Anesthesiology and Acute Pain Medicine Fellowship Directors Group (2011) Guidelines for fellowship training in Regional Anesthesiology and Acute Pain Medicine: Second Edition, 2010. Reg Anesth Pain Med 36:282-288.
11. Sites BD, Chan VW, Neal JM et al (2010) The American Society of Regional Anesthesia and Pain Medicine and the European Society of Regional Anaesthesia and Pain Therapy joint committee recommendations for education and training in ultrasound-guided regional anesthesia. Reg Anesth Pain Med. 35:S74-S80.
12. Hargett MJ, Beckman JD, Liguori GA et al (2005) Education Committee in the Department of Anesthesiology at Hospital for Special Surgery. Guidelines for regional anesthesia fellowship training. Reg Anesth Pain Med 30:218-225.
13. Smith HM, Kopp SL, Jacob AK et al (2009) Designing and implementing a comprehensive learner-centered regional anesthesia curriculum. Reg Anesth Pain Med 34:88-894.
14. Hocking G, Hebard S, Mitchell CH (2011) A review of the benefits and pitfalls of phantoms in ultrasound-guided regional anesthesia. Reg Anesth Pain Med. 36:162-170.
15. Giaufre E, Dalens B, Gombert A (1996) Epidemiology and morbidity of regional anesthesia in children: a one-year prospective survey of the French-Language Society of Pediatric Anesthesiologists. Anesth Analg 83:904-912.
16. Ecoffey C, Lacroix F, Giaufre E et al (2010) Epidemiology and morbidity of regional anesthesia in children: a follow-up one-year prospective survey of the French-Language Society of Paediatric Anaesthesiologists (ADARPEF). Paediatr Anaesth 20:1061-1069.
17. Polaner DM, Walker BJ, Taenzer A et al (2012) Pediatric Regional Anesthesia Network: a multi-institutional study of the use and incidence of complications of pediatric regional anesthesia. Anesth Analg (in press)
18. Rubin K, Sullivan D, Sadhasivam S (2009) Are peripheral and neuraxial blocks with ultrasound guidance more effective and safe in children? Paediatr Anaesth. 19:92-96.
19. Walker IA, Newton M, Bosenberg AT (2011) Improving surgical safety globally: pulse oximetry and the WHO Guidelines for Safe Surgery. Paediatr Anaesth. 21:825-828.
20. Special themed issue: Pediatric Regional Anaesthesia. (2012) Lonnqvist PA Guest Ed Paediatr Anaesth 22(1):1-118.
21. Suresh S, Voronov P (2012) Head and neck blocks in infants, children, and adolescents. Paediatr Anaesth. 22:81-87.
22. Tsui BC, Suresh S (2010) Ultrasound imaging for regional anesthesia in infants, children, and adolescents: a review of current literature and its application in the practice of neuraxial blocks. Anesthesiology. 112:719-728.
23. Tsui B, Suresh S (2010) Ultrasound imaging for regional anesthesia in infants, children, and adolescents: a review of current literature and its application in the practice of extremity and trunk blocks. Anesthesiology 112:473-492.
24. Mesnil M, Dadure C, Captier G et al (2010) A new approach for peri-operative analgesia of cleft palate repair in infants: the bilateral suprazygomatic maxillary nerve block. Paediatr Anaesth. 20:343-349.

25. Sola C, Raux O, Savath L et al (2012) Ultrasound guidance characteristics and efficiency of suprazygomatic maxillary nerve blocks in infants: a descriptive prospective study. Paediatr Anaesth. May 15 [Epub ahead of print]
26. Palmer GM, Luk VH, Smith KR et al (2011) Audit of initial use of the ultrasound-guided transversus abdominis plane block in children. Anaesth Intensive Care. 39:279-286.
27. Walker BJ, Flack SH, Bosenberg AT (2011) Predicting lumbar plexus depth in children and adolescents. Anesth Analg 112:661-665.
28. Dadure C, Raux O, Gaudard Pet al (2004) Continuous psoas compartment blocks after major orthopedic surgery in children: a prospective computed tomographic scan and clinical studies. Anesth Analg 98:623-628.
29. Dadure C, Raux O, Gaudard P et al (2004) Continuous psoas compartment blocks after major orthopedic surgery in children: a prospective computed tomographic scan and clinical studies Anesth Analg. 98:623-628.
30. Ponde VC, Desai AP, Shah DM et al (2011) Feasibility and efficacy of placement of continuous sciatic perineural catheters solely under ultrasound guidance in children: a descriptive study. Paediatr Anaesth. 21:406-410
31. Dobereiner EF, Cox RG, Ewen A et al (2010) Evidence-based clinical update: Which local anesthetic drug for pediatric caudal block provides optimal efficacy with the fewest side effects? Can J Anaesth 57:1102-1110.
32. Lonnqvist PA (2005) Adjuncts to caudal block in children: quovadis? Br J Anaesth 95, 431-433
33. Disma N, Frawley G, Mameli L et al (2011) Effect of epidural clonidine on minimum local anesthetic concentration (ED50) of levobupivacaine for caudal block in children. Paediatr Anaesth 21:128-135.
34. Schnabel A, Poepping DM, Pogatzki-Zahn EM et al (2011) Efficacy and safety of clonidine as additive for caudal regional anesthesia: a quantitative systematic review of randomized controlled trials. Paediatr Anaesth 21:1219-1230
35. Schnabel A, Poepping DM, Kranke P et al (2011) Efficacy and adverse effects of ketamine as an additive for paediatric caudal anaesthesia: a quantitative systematic review of randomized controlled trials. Br J Anaesth 107:601-611.
36. Menzies R, Congreve K, Herodes V et al (2009) A survey of pediatric caudal extradural anesthesia practice. Paediatr Anaesth 19:829-836.
37. Akin A, Ocalan S, Esmaoglu A et al (2010) The effects of caudal or intravenous clonidine on postoperative analgesia produced by caudal levobupivacaine in children. Paediatr Anaesth 20:350-355
38. McCartney CJL, Duggan E, Apatu E (2007) Should we add clonidine to local anesthetic for peripheral nerve blockade? A qualitative systematic review of the literature. Regional Anesthesia Pain Medicine 32:330-338
39. Trifa M, Ben Khalifa S, Jendoubi A et al (2012) Clonidine does not improve quality of ropivacaine axillary brachial plexus block in children. Paediatr Anaesth. 22:425-9.
40. Lönnqvist PA (2012) Alpha-2 adrenoceptor agonists as adjuncts to Peripheral Nerve Blocks in Children - is there a mechanism of action and should we use them? Paediatr Anaesth 22:421-424.

Drugs and Clinical Pharmacology of Central Blocks in Infants and Children

12

Per-Arne Lönnqvist

12.1 Drugs and Clinical Pharmacology of Central Blocks in Infants and Children

Even though more than 100 years have passed since the first description of the use of central blocks in children (Bier, 1899, Tyrell-Gray, 1909), there are still new and important things to learn within this particular field of anesthesia. Therefore, to perform safe and effective regional anesthesia in infants and children, a solid knowledge of the age-related pharmacology of both local anesthetics and their adjuncts is an absolute prerequisite. Although not as extensive as in adults, the published literature within the field of clinical pharmacology of local anesthetics and their adjuncts in infants and children is quite substantial at this point in time.

To avoid redundant publications and the repetition of already published material within this field, I have refrained from producing yet another text on this topic. Instead, the current chapter provides a synopsis of the current knowledge and incorporates the reproduction of a review article by Professor Jean-Xavier Mazoit, titled *Local Anesthetics and their Adjuncts*, which was recently published in *Pediatric Anesthesia* (http://onlinelibrary.wiley.com/doi/10.1111/j.1460-9592.2011.03692.x/pdf). This has been made possible by the kind permission of Professor Mazoit, the editor-in-chief Neil Morton, and by Wiley-Blackwell Publishing Ltd. For information on the toxicity aspects, the reader is referred to another review from the same themed issue of *Pediatric Anesthesia* [1] (works cited in paragraph 12.1 have been kept separately in the first group of references listed at the end of the chapter).

Following the publication of the review article reproduced herein, further information and discussion has been published with regard to the use of ketamine as an adjunct in newborns and infants. Thus, in rodent experiments, Walker and colleagues have been able to show that the application of clinically relevant doses of

P.-A. Lönnqvist (✉)
Department of Physiology and Pharmacology, Section of Anesthesiology and Intensive Care
The Karolinska Institute, Stockholm, Sweden
e-mail: per-arne.lonnqvist@ki.se

M. Astuto (ed.) *Pediatric Anesthesia, Intensive Care and Pain: Standardization in Clinical Practice*. Anesthesia, Intensive Care and Pain in Neonates and Children
DOI: 10.1007/978-88-470-2685-8_12, © Springer-Verlag Italia 2013

intrathecal ketamine in young rodents does result in apoptosis of spinal neurons as previously shown for cortical neurons [2]. This is in sharp contrast to findings from similar studies for morphine and clonidine, both appearing to be associated with a comfortable margin of safety with regard to programmed spinal cord cell death [3,4]. Based on these findings, a recent editorial in the *British Journal of Anaesthesia* questioned the use of ketamine as an adjunct to caudal and epidural blocks in newborns and infants and instead recommended the use of clonidine in a situation when an adjunct drug is deemed necessary in this age group [5].

Therefore, the key points are:

1. Due to the reduced toxicity risk compared to racemic bupivacaine, the regular use of ropivacaine or levobupivacaine is advocated in infants and children (with the exception of intrathecal blockade).

2. There is little evidence for the efficacy of the use of opioids as adjuncts to central blocks in children (with the exception of preservative-free morphine). Within this context, it should also be remembered that opioids, apart from being associated with a risk of respiratory depression, are also associated with a number of less serious but still very distressing side effects (e.g., postoperative nausea and vomiting, pruritus, urinary retention, and interference with gastrointestinal motility) [6].

3. For a single-injection caudal block in children above 1 year of age, the use of ketamine appears the most effective adjunct in prolonging the duration of the block.

4. Clonidine is associated with a good safety profile and can be used as an adjunct drug in all age groups. It can also be used as an adjunct for both central and peripheral nerve blocks [7].

5. The use of adjuncts other than preservative-free solutions of clonidine, ketamine, and morphine must still be seen as experimental and should not be used routinely [8].

When reading the review by Professor Mazoit which follows, the reader should be mindful of a typographical error. With regard to the dosing of the lipid rescue, mL (milliliters) rather than mg (milligrams), should have been used throughout. The initial dose of Intralipid is 2–5 mL/kg^{-1} and can be repeated up to a total of 10 mL/kg^{-1}, rather than 10 mg/kg^{-1}.

12.2 Local Anesthetics and Their Adjuncts: A Review Article by Jean-Xavier Mazoit

Local anesthetics (LA) block propagation of impulses along nerve fibers by inactivation of voltage-gated sodium channels, which initiate action potentials [1]. They act on the cytosolic side of phospholipid membranes. Two main chemical compounds are used, amino esters and amino amides. Amino esters are degraded by pseudocholinesterases in plasma. Aminoamides are metabolized exclusively by the liver. Only amide LAs will be considered in this article.

12.2.1 Pharmacokinetics

Local anesthetics (LAs) are small molecules with molecular weights ranging from 220 to 288 [2]. They contain an aromatic ring, an intermediate chain (amide group), and a hydrophilic residue with a tertiary amine. They are weak bases with pKas between 7.6 (mepivacaine) and 8.1 (bupivacaine and ropivacaine). At a pH of 7.40, 60–85% of the molecules are ionized and diffuse in hydric compartments. LAs are also soluble in lipids and then easily cross cell membranes. Bupivacaine is ten times more liposoluble than lidocaine; ropivacaine is four times as soluble as lidocaine (partition coefficient from XlogP) (Table 12.1). With the exception of lidocaine, all amide LAs possess an asymmetric carbon. Although the physiochemical properties (pKa, distribution coefficient) of the isomers are identical, the enantiomers have different affinities for the biological effectors (channels, receptors, proteins) [3]. Ropivacaine and levobupivacaine are pure S-(−) enantiomers. LAs are marketed as hydrochloride salts in water at pH of 4–5 to prevent them from precipitation [4]. Plain solutions of amide LAs are preservative-free; only epinephrine-containing solutions include metabisulfite.

Table 12.1 Physicochemical properties of local anesthetics

Drug	Molecular weight[a] (Da)	pKa[b]	Partition[c] coefficient	Protein binding (%)	Onset of action	Duration of action	Potency[d]
Amides							
Lidocaine	234	7.8	234	65	Short	1 h 30 min–2 h	1
Prilocaine	220	8.0	126	55	Short	1 h 30 min–2 h	1
Mepivacaine	246	7.7	79	75	Short	1 h 30 min–2 h	1
Bupivacaine[e]	288	8.1	2512	95	Intermediate	3 h–3 h 30 min	4
Ropivacaine	274	8.1	794	96	Intermediate	2 h 30 min–3 h	3.3

[a] Free base.
[b] pKa at 37°C.
[c] Octanol/buffer partition calculated from XlogP.
[d] Potency is relative to lidocaine.
[e] Levobupivacaine has similar physicochemical properties with a slightly lower potency.

12.2.1.1 Binding to Blood Components

Amide LAs distribute in red cells (20–30% depending on the hematocrit) and bind to serum proteins [2,5]. Like most weak bases, amide LAs bind to both a1-acid glycoprotein (AGP) and to human serum albumin (HSA). The stereospecificity of this binding is insignificant, at least on a clinical point of view [6]. Despite its low concentration in serum (< 1 g/L^{-1} in adults), AGP is the major protein that binds LAs. AGP concentration is very low at birth and progressively increases during the first year of life [5,7]. It is why neonates and young infants have a much higher free fraction of LAs than adults. AGP is an acute phase protein, and its concentration increases rapidly in inflammatory states like in the postoperative period [7]. LAs also bind to HSA, but with a very low affinity. It is only because HSA is the most abundant protein in serum that its binding capacity is significant.

12.2.1.2 Absorption

After applying topical anesthesia to the upper airway, LAs are rapidly absorbed. This may induce toxicity, particularly in young children. This is why it is important to use nozzles that deliver no more than 10 mg with each squeeze [8]. The EMLA (Eutectic Mixture of Local Anesthetics) cream is absorbed in significant amounts in premature babies and neonates [9]. The cream contains prilocaine, which produces methemoglobinemia in neonates and infants, especially if they are also treated with trimethoprim-sulfamethoxazole [10]. The efficacy of the cream has been questioned in premature babies because of a high skin blood flow [9].

After injection, amide LAs have a bioavailability of one (metabolism is exclusively hepatic) [11]. They bind to tissues, which delays their absorption. This delay varies depending on the site of injection. In adults, 3 h after an epidural injection, only 70% of a dose of lidocaine and 50% of a dose of bupivacaine or of ropivacaine are absorbed, which are safety factors [11]. From adult studies, it is clear that the speed of drug absorption decreases from head to foot and from the thoracic to the caudal portion of the epidural space. Lidocaine and bupivacaine concentrations peak about 30 min after caudal or lumbar injection in infants and adults [5,12–17]. The Tmax for ropivacaine is much longer in infants than in children [18,19] and possibly in children than in adults [18–26]. CYP1A2, which metabolizes lidocaine and ropivacaine, is immature before 4–7 years of age [27].

Levobupivacaine is principally metabolized by the CYP3A4/7, which has full enzymatic capacity by the age of 1 year [28].

12.2.1.3 Distribution

The volume of distribution of LAs at steady state (V_{ss}) is slightly < 1 L/kg^{-1} (Table 12.2) [5,11–26]. Because of delayed drug absorption leading to the 'flip-flop' effect,[1] terminal half-lives and volumes calculated after non-intravenous (i.v.) routes of administration are markedly overestimated [11,20,29–31]. Only total body clearance of the drug is measured accurately following extravascular administration (but sampling must take place over a prolonged period of time). It is highly probable that LAs distribute in a larger volume in neonates and in infants than in adults, thus preventing high serum drug concentrations from occurring after a single injection, but not following several injections. The volume of distribution of ropivacaine is smaller than that of bupivacaine in adults and probably in pediatric patients [2].

12.2.1.4 Elimination

All amide LAs are metabolized by the liver cytochrome P450 enzymes. Bupivacaine is predominantly metabolized into pipecoloxylidide (PPX) by CYP3A4/7 [28]. Ropivacaine is predominantly metabolized to 3'- and 4'-OH-ropivacaine by CYP1A2

---

[1] Because compartmental pharmacokinetics are based on the assumption of linearity, concentration is described by a sum of exponentials with the assumption that absorption is faster than distribution and distribution is faster than elimination. If absorption is longer than elimination, it is not possible to distinguish between the phases. In other words, if absorption continues during elimination, the terminal phase appears falsely prolonged.

Table 12.2 Bupivacaine, levobupivacaine, and ropivacaine pharmacokinetics after different routes in infants and children compared with adults

	Free fraction	V_{ss}^{a} (L/kg^{-1})	CLT/f (mL/min^{-1}/kg^{-1})	CLU/f (mL/min^{1}/kg^{-1})	T1/2^{a} (h)
Bupivacaine					
i.v. adults	0.05	0.85–1.3	4.5–8.1	100	1.8
Epidural adults			4–5.6		5.1–10.6
Infants caudal single shot children	0.16 (0.05–0.35)	3.9	7.1		
(5–10 years)		2.7	10		
Infants epidural	(0.06–0.24)[b]		5.5–7.5[b]	36–73	
prolonged	(0.03–0.18)[c]		3.5–4[c]	36–73	
Levobupivacaine					
i.v. adults	0.045	0.72	4.2	116	2.6
Caudal, infants 0.6–2.9 months	0.13	2.87	6.28	51.7	
Ropivacaine					
i.v. adults	0.05	0.5–0.6	4.2–5.3	100	1.7
Epidural adults			4.0–5.7	70	2.9–5.4
Caudal single shot					
Neonates	0.07			50–58	
Infants	0.05–0.10	2.1	5.2		
Children	5.2 (1.3–7.3)	2.4	7.4	151	
Epidural prolonged					
Neonates		2.4	4.26		
Infants		2.4	6.15		
Children	0.04		8.5	220	

Vss, volume of distribution at steady state, *CLU/f,* total body clearance over bioavailability (*T*, total fraction; *U*, unbound fraction), *T1/2*, terminal half-life.

For adults, a mean body weight (BW) of 75 kg has been assumed. Injections are overestimated because of a flip-flop effect (i.e., because absorption last longer than elimination).

[a]Apparent value, T1/2 and volumes measured after non-i.v.

[b]After 3-h infusion.

[c]After 48-h infusion, CLT decreases with time because protein binding increases.

and to a minor extent to PPX by CYP3A4 [27]. These enzymes are not fully mature at birth and have important differences in their developmental expression. Contrary to lidocaine, bupivacaine and ropivacaine have a relatively low hepatic extraction ratio (0.30–0.35) and are considered rate limited for their elimination. Thus, the intrinsic hepatic clearance and the free fraction are the major determinants of total clearance. After surgery, serum AGP concentrations increase, which increases protein binding. A parallel decrease in total clearance is observed [7]. However, this only leads to a resetting in total serum concentration, and the unbound concentration remains constant. Bupivacaine clearance is low at birth and increases slightly during the first 6–9 months of life (Fig. 12.1). Ropivacaine clearance, which

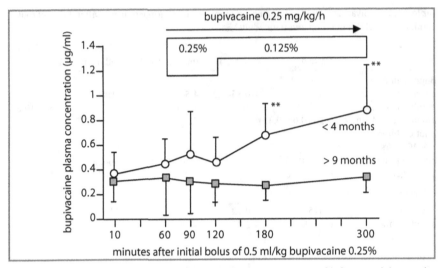

Fig. 12.1 Bupivacaine plasma concentrations measured in two groups of infants receiving continuous bupivacaine infusion by the caudal route for postoperative analgesia. Dosing was calculated to maintain steady concentrations in the older patients (> 9 months old). The bupivacaine concentrations increased with infusion time in the younger infants (< 4 months old), thus demonstrating that clearance was markedly lower in the younger patients. Reproduced from Luz G, Innerhofer I, Bachmann B et al. Bupivacaine plasma concentrations during continuous epidural anesthesia in infants and children. Anesth Analg 1996; 82: 231–234. February 1, Lippincott Williams & Wilkins [78]

is also low in neonates and infants, increases during the first 2–6 years of life [19]. This is likely the cause of the delayed ropivacaine Cmax observed in the younger patients after caudal injection.

Concentrations leading to toxicity are largely unknown. In adult volunteers, the threshold of toxicity is about 0.2–0.3 mg/L^{-1} of unbound bupivacaine and 0.4–0.6 mg/L^{-1} of unbound ropivacaine or levobupivacaine [32–35]. Neonates and infants seem to be more prone to develop toxicity [36,37] because of a higher serum free fraction, a lower clearance, and an increased susceptibility to cardiac toxicity. During prolonged administration of LAs for postoperative pain relief, it is assumed that the intrinsic unbound clearance is unaffected during the whole period of administration and the unbound concentration reaches a steady level 12–18 h after the initiation of infusion. Because of the inflammatory process leading to increased serum binding capacity, the plasma concentrations of total (levo) bupivacaine and ropivacaine tend to increase postoperatively during more than 2–4 days.

12.2.2 Pharmacodynamics

Local anesthetics block the propagation of impulses along nerve fibers because of the inactivation of voltage-gated sodium channels. LAs cross membranes as free bases (unionized). Inside the cells, they become ionized and bind to specific amino acids within the channel pore, thus mechanically blocking the pore [1]. LAs also block potassium and calcium channels at slightly higher drug concentrations than those needed to block sodium channels [38,39]. Voltage-gated potassium channels initiate repolarization in the nerve. In the myocardium, some of these channels [including the human ether-à-go-go related gene (hERG) channel] are responsible for genetically induced arrhythmias, such as the long-QT, short-QT, or Brugada syndromes. These channels are blocked by LA concentrations just slightly higher than those needed to block sodium channels [38,39]. Unlike the central nervous system (CNS) and heart, peripheral nerves only express a small number of potassium channels. Both sodium and potassium channel blockades are stereospecific [38–40]. The S enantiomers induce less block than R enantiomers. LAs bind to the myocardial ryanodine receptor and L-type calcium channels [41,42], but it is unclear if blockade of these channels affect the cardiotoxicity of long-lasting LAs.

Nerve fibers are either myelinated or unmyelinated. After initial depolarization, the sodium channels become unreceptive to stimulation (refractory period), which prevents backward propagation of impulses. The action potential of unmyelinated fibers propagates continuously.

Myelin insulates myelinated fibers, and this layer is interrupted regularly by the nodes of Ranvier. The sudden depolarization of the node induces an electrical field, which extends to 2–3 nodes. Action potentials "jump" rapidly from one node to the next. Because the distance between nodes is greater in heavily myelinated fibers (there are 3–4 nodes per cm in Aa fibers and 20–30 nodes per cm in Ad fibers), the conduction velocity is faster in motor than in small sensory fibers and faster in small sensory fibers than in high threshold fibers that conduct pain signals [43]. Small unmyelinated or lightly myelinated fibers–the fibers that conduct pain signals–are blocked by lower concentrations of drug and during a longer period of time than heavily myelinated fibers. Myelinization begins during the third trimester of pregnancy and is incomplete at birth. After birth, myelinization increases rapidly and is almost complete by 3–4 years of age [44,45]. In rats, the nodes of Ranvier are fully mature at 2–3 weeks of age. Interestingly, the internode distance is similar between 2-week-old and adult rats. This may explain why infants and young children need larger volumes per kg of LAs than older children or adults (Fig. 12.2) [46].

Fortunately, the concentration of LA needed to cause the block is lower. Surprisingly, infants require larger doses of LAs for spinal anesthesia, and the duration of the spinal block is shorter. Some authors have attributed this difference to larger volumes and a more rapid turnover of cerebrospinal fluid (CSF) in neonates and infants than in older children and adults. However, MRI studies have shown that the CSF volume and CSF turnover are lower in neonates and infants than in children and adults [47,48]. The major factor responsible for this short effect seems to depend on the number of nodes of Ranvier blocked because the distance between nodes is fixed soon after birth [44,45].

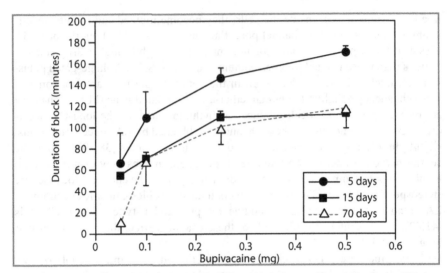

Fig. 12.2 Duration of sciatic nerve motor block in infant rats according to the dose of bupivacaine used. Rats aged 5 days had a prolonged block as compared to the other two groups. Two-week¬-old rats had a similar duration of block as compared to 10-week-old rats despite an 8–10 times difference in body weight: The same dose gave the same duration of block likely because the internode distance is fixed after the age of 1–2 weeks [drawn from the data of Kohane DS, Sankar WN, Shubina M et al. Sciatic nerve blockade in infant, adolescent, and adult rats: a comparison of ropivacaine with bupivacaine. Anesthesiology 1998; 89: 1199–1208. November, Lippincott Williams & Wilkins [46]

12.2.2.1 Effects on the Central Nervous System and Cardiovascular System

Like all inhibitors of sodium channels, LAs possess anticonvulsive effects at low dosage, which is why lidocaine is still used to treat intractable epilepsy in neonates and infants [49]. At higher doses, LAs induce convulsions and coma. However, the therapeutic ratio is low. In similar concentrations to those that cause convulsions, long-lasting LAs can induce cardiac arrhythmias. With the exception of nodal conduction, which depends on calcium channels, conduction in the heart depends on sodium channels. LAs prolong the refractory period, but the balance between the increase in effective refractory period and the decrease in the ventricular conduction velocity does not favor LAs. Long-lasting LAs, like bupivacaine, profoundly decrease ventricular conduction velocity [50–52]. This phenomenon is markedly amplified by tachycardia–it is the phasic block. Because neonates and infants have higher heart rates than adults, they are likely more sensitive to LA-induced blocks than adults. LAs also impair myocardial contractility but without any stereospecificity [52]. The S enantiomers (ropivacaine and levobupivacaine) have mild vasoconstrictive properties.

12.2.2.2 Stereospecificity

Mepivacaine, prilocaine, bupivacaine, and ropivacaine have an asymmetric carbon. Protein binding, pharmacokinetics, and nerve blocks have little stereoselectivity, which is why levobupivacaine has almost the same blocking properties as its racemic counterpart. In the heart, the effect on cardiac conduction is stereospecific (ropivacaine and levobupivacaine induce much less block than their corresponding R (+) enantiomer or the racemic mixture), whereas contractility is unaffected by stereoselectivity [51,52].

LAs have anti-inflammatory properties and inhibit platelet aggregation [53], decrease leukocyte priming and the production of free radicals [54–56]. Systemically administered lidocaine has antinociceptive effects, particularly on neuropathic pain [57]. Consequently, LAs are now used preoperatively to prevent postoperative hyperalgesia in adults [58]. Interestingly, LAs can prevent and even treat complex regional pain syndrome in adults and children by limiting the neuropathic inflammatory processes [59,60].

12.2.2.3 Toxicity of Local Anesthetics

At the site of injection, the minimum concentration required to produce a nerve blockade is 300–1500 µM for lidocaine and 100–500 µM for bupivacaine [61]. These concentrations (in the millimolar range) impair mitochondrial function and may be responsible for the observed nerve and muscle toxicity. Care should be taken when regional anesthesia is provided for eye surgery in adults, for children with myopathies (bupivacaine is an *in vitro* model of Duchene's myopathy), and perhaps for children with mitochondrial cytopathy [62,63]. With that respect, the site of injection for central blocks is far from any muscle.

After both local and regional anesthesia, neurological or cardiac toxicity related to excessive blood concentration may occur [64,65]. Because of their low protein binding and intrinsic clearance, infants are more prone to LA toxicity than adults. General anesthesia may conceal the early signs of LA toxicity in children. In addition to pharmacokinetic factors, the rapid heart rate of children may increase the risk of cardiac toxicity induced by LA toxicity. Ropivacaine and levobupivacaine [S-())-enantiomers] are less toxic than racemic bupivacaine [32–35]. Even if toxic events occur with ropivacaine, small doses of epinephrine should produce rapid recovery. Impaired ventricular conduction is the primary manifestation of LA toxicity. QRS widening, bradycardia, and torsades de pointe are followed by either ventricular fibrillation and/or asystole [65]. The slight decrease in myocardial contractility caused by LAs is usually not a major problem. Treatment includes oxygenation, cardiac massage, and epinephrine, which is given in small incremental boluses beginning with $1–2$ µg/kg^{-1} [66]. If ventricular fibrillation persists, defibrillation ($2–4$ J/kg^{-1}) is performed. Although resuscitation measures must be initiated immediately, the specific treatment of LA toxicity is rapid administration of Intralipid (Kabivitrum Inc., Stockholm, Sweden). Numerous case reports have shown that rapid bolus injections of a lipid emulsion reverse the toxic effects of LAs [66–69]. Because 1 mole of Intralipid (Kabivitrum Inc.) binds > 3000 times more molecules of bupivacaine than a mole of buffer, the volume of distribution suddenly increases [70]. The recommended dose of 20% Intralipid (Kabivitrum Inc.) for pediatric patients is $2–5$ mL/kg^{-1} by i.v. bolus. If cardiac function does not return, this dose (up to 10 mg/kg^{-1}) is repeated. The lipid emulsion decreases LA elimination; thus, the cardiac effects may recur later.

12.2.2.4 Adjuvants

Adjuvants are often used to prolong the duration of analgesia.

Adrenaline (5 µg/mL^{-1} = 1/200,000) decreases bupivacaine Cmax, without affecting the time to peak concentration. In < 6-month-old infants, 2.5 µg/mL^{-1} 1/400,000 epinephrine has been recommended [71]. However, the drug is less efficacious with long-acting S-()- enantiomers and has limited use with these solutions. Plain solutions of LAs must be used for penile, interdigital, and eye blocks. Adrenaline also slightly increases the duration of postoperative analgesia after caudal anesthesia. Clonidine 1–2 µg/kg^{-1}, either i.v. or in the epidural space, prolongs the duration of caudal blocks [72]. Clonidine also enhances the efficacy of dilute long-acting agents (e.g., 0.1% ropivacaine). More than 2 g/kg^{-1} may lead to hypotension.

Clonidine is not recommended for infants < 3 months of age because it can cause apnea in this age group. It has been shown that clonidine injected i.v. has a similar effect than when epidurally injected [73].

Ketamine is also used as an adjuvant for epidural block [74]. The pure preservative-free S(+) ketamine is preferable because it is less toxic for the nervous structures than the racemic mixture. However, some authors recommend avoiding the use of ketamine because of its potential toxicity [75,76]. The usual dose injected caudally is 1 and 0.5 mg/kg^{-1} for the S(+) and racemic ketamine, respectively.

Opioids are often used as adjuvants for epidural block. After 6–9 months of age, adding opioids to LAs prolongs epidural analgesia for up to 24 h. Hydrophobic agents (fentanyl, sufentanil) must be placed at the metameric level where the pain will occur [77]. Preservative-free morphine easily spreads rostrally and can be placed at a lower metameric level. The bolus dose of morphine is 25–30 µg/kg^{-1} in the epidural space, which is followed by a continuous infusion of 1 µg/kg^{-1}/h^{-1}. When continuous epidural administration of fentanyl or sufentanil is combined with LAs, the doses are 0.2 and 0.1 µg/kg^{-1}/h^{-1}, respectively. Morphine 5–10 µg/kg^{-1} can be used as the sole agent for spinal analgesia during general anesthesia. In case of urinary retention, naloxone 1 µg/kg^{-1} or nalbuphine 0.1 mg/kg^{-1} can be injected as an i.v bolus. An i.v. bolus of naloxone 1–2 µg/kg^{-1} followed by a continuous infusion of 1–2 µg/kg^{-1}/h^{-1} is usually efficacious in case of pruritus.

References

1. Lönnqvist PA (2012) Toxicity of local anesthetic drugs: a pediatric perspective. Paediatr Anaesth 22:39-43
2. Walker SM, Westin BD, Deumens R et al (2010) Effects of Intrathecal Ketamine in the Neonatal Rat: Evaluation of Apoptosis and Long-term Functional Outcome. Anesthesiology 113:147-159
3. Westin BD, Walker SM, Deumens R et al (2010) Validation of a Preclinical Spinal Safety Model: Effects of Intrathecal Morphine in the Neonatal Rat. Anesthesiology 113:183-199

4. Walker SM, Grafe M, Yaksh TL (2012) Intrathecal clonidine in the neonatal rat: dose-dependent analgesia and evaluation of spinal apoptosis and toxicity. Anest Analg 2012; in press
5. Lönnqvist PA, Walker SM (2012) Ketamine as an adjunct to caudal blockade in neonates and infants: is it time to re-evaluate? Br J Anaesth 2012; in press
6. Lönnqvist PA, Ivani G, Moriarty T (2002) Use of caudal-epidural opioids in children: still state of the art or the beginning of the end? Paediatr Anaesth 12:747-749.
7. Lönnqvist PA (2012) Alpha-2 adrenoceptor agonists as adjuncts to Peripheral Nerve Blocks in Children–is there a mechanism of action and should we use them? Paediatr Anaesth 22:421-424
8. Lönnqvist PA(2005) Adjuncts to caudal block in children – Quo vadis? Br J Anaesth 95:431-433

References of the Review Article

1. Catterall WA (2002) Molecular mechanisms of gating and drug block of sodium channels. Novartis Found Symp 241:206-218
2. Mazoit JX, Dalens BJ (2004) Pharmacokinetics of local anaesthetics in infants and children. Clin Pharmacokinet 43:17-32
3. Nau C, Strichartz GR (2002) Drug chirality in anesthesia. Anesthesiology 97:497-502
4. Cartwright PD, Fyhr P (1988) The manufacture and storage of local anesthetics. Reg Anesth 13:1-12
5. Mazoit JX, Denson DD, Samii K (1988) Pharmacokinetics of bupivacaine following caudal anesthesia in infants. Anesthesiology 68:387-391
6. Mazoit JX, Denson DD, Samii K (1996) Pharmaisolated albumin and isolated alpha-1-acid glycoprotein. Differences between the two enantiomers are partly due to cooperativity. J Pharmacol Exp Ther 276:109-115
7. Meunier JF, Goujard E, Dubousset AM et al (2001) Pharmacokinetics of bupivacaine after continuous epidural infusion in infants with and without biliary atresia. Anesthesiology 95:87-95
8. Sitbon P, Laffon M, Lesage V et al (1997) Lidocaine plasma concentrations in pediatric patients after providing airway topical anesthesia from a calibrated device. Anesth Russell SC, Doyle E. A risk-benefit assessment of topical percutaneous local anaesthetics in children. Drug Saf 16:279-287
9. Taddio A, Ohlsson A, Einarson TR et al (1998) A systematic review of lidocaine-prilocaine cream (EMLA) in the treatment of acute pain in neonates. Pediatrics 101:E1
10. Russell SC, Doyle E (1997) A risk-benefit assessment of topical percutaneous local anaesthetics in children. Drug Saf 16:279-287
11. Burm AGL (1989) Clinical pharmacokinetics of epidural and spinal anesthesia. Clin Pharmacokinet 16:283-311
12. Ecoffey C, Desparmet J, Berdeaux A et al (1984) Pharmacokinetics of lidocaine in children following caudal anaesthesia. Br J Anaesth 56:1399-1402
13. Ecoffey C, Desparmet J, Berdeaux A et al (2004) Bupivacaine in children: pharmacokinetics children under 2 years of age. Br J Anaesth 92:218-222
14. Chalkiadis GA, Eyres RL, Cranswick N et al (2004) Pharmacokinetics of levobupivacaine 0.25% following caudal administration in children under 2 years of age. Br J Anaesth 92:218-222
15. Cortínez LI, Fuentes R, Solari S et al (2008) Pharmacokinetics of levobupivacaine (2.5 mg/kg) after caudal administration in children younger than 3 years. Anesth Analg 107:1182-1184
16. Desparmet J, Meistelman C, Barre J et al (1987) Continuous epidural infusion of bupivacaine for postoperative pain relief in children. Anesthesiology 67:108-110

17. Lerman J, Nolan J, Eyres R et al (2003) Efficacy, safety, and pharmacokinetics of levobupivacaine with and without fentanyl after continuous epidural infusion in children: a multicenter trial. Anesthesiology 99:1166-1174

18. Ala-Kokko TI, Partanen A, Karinen J et al (2000) Pharmacokinetics of 0.2% ropivacaine and 0.2% bupivacaine following caudal blocks in children. Acta Anaesthesiol Scand 44:1099-1102

19. Lonnqvist PA, Westrin P, Larsson BA et al (2000) Ropivacaine pharmacokinetics after caudal block in 1-8 year old children. Br J Anaesth 85:506-511

20. Emanuelsson BM, Persson J, Sandin S et al (1997) Intraindividual and interindividual variability in the disposition of the local anesthetic ropivacaine in healthy subjects. Ther Drug Monit 19:126-131

21. Hansen TG, Ilett KF, Reid C et al (2001) Caudal ropivacaine in infants: population pharmacokinetics and plasma concentrations. Anesthesiology 94:579-584

22. McCann ME, Sethna NF, Mazoit JX et al (2001) The pharmacokinetics of epidural ropivacaine in infants and young children. Anesth Analg 93:893-897

23. Bösenberg AT, Thomas J, Cronje L et al (1998) Pharmacokinetics and efficacy of ropivavoxamine and ketoconazole as in vivo inhibitors. Clin Pharmacol Ther 64:484-491

24. Rapp HJ, Molnar V, Austin S et al (2004) Ropivacaine in neonates and infants: a population pharmacokinetic evaluation following single caudal block. Pediatr Anesth 14:724-732

25. Berde CB, Yaster M, Meretoja O et al (2008) Stable plasma concentrations of unbound ropivacaine during postoperative epidural infusion for 24-72 hours in children. Eur J Anaesthesiol 25:410-417

26. Dalens B, Ecoffey C, Joly A et al (2001) Pharmacokinetics and analgesic effect of ropivacaine following ilioinguinal/iliohypogastric nerve block in children. Paediatr Anaesth 11:415-420

27. Arlander E, Ekstrom G, Alm C et al (1998) Metabolism of ropivacaine in humans is mediated by CYP1A2 and to a minor extent by CYP3A4: an interaction study with fluvoxamine and ketoconazole as in vivo inhibitors. Clin Pharmacol Ther 64:484-491

28. Gantenbein M, Attolini L, Bruguerolle B et al (2000) Oxidative metabolism of bupivacaine into pipecolylxylidine in humans is mainly catalyzed by CYP3A. Drug Metab Dispos 28:383-385

29. Burm AG, van der Meer AD, van Kleef JW et al (1994) Pharmacokinetics of the enantiomers of bupivacaine following intravenous administration of the racemate. Br J Clin Pharmacol 38:125-129

30. Burm AGL, Vermeulen NPE, Van Kleef JW et al (1987) Pharmacokinetics of lidocaine and bupivacaine in surgical patients following epidural administration. Simultaneous investigation of absorption and disposition kinetics using stable isotopes. Clin Pharmacokinet 13:191-203

31. Burm AG, Stienstra R, Brouwer RP et al (2000) Epidural infusion of ropivacaine for postoperative analgesia after major orthopedic surgery: pharmacokinetic evaluation. Anesthesiology 93:395-403

32. Scott DB, Lee A, Fagan D et al (1989) Acute toxic ity of ropivacaine compared with that of bupivacaine. Anesth Analg 69:563-569

33. Knudsen K, Beckman Suurkü la M, Blomberg S et al (1997) Central nervous and cardiovascular effects of i.v. infusions of ropivacaine, bupivacaine and placebo in volunteers. Br J Anaesth 78:507-514

34. Bardsley H, Gristwood R, Baker H et al (1998) A comparison of the cardiovascular effects of levobupivacaine and rac-bupivacaine following intravenous administration to healthy volunteers. Br J Clin Pharmacol 46:245-249

35. Stewart J, Kellett N, Castro D (1995) The central nervous system and cardiovascular effects of levobupivacaine and ropivacaine in healthy tricular myocytes. Circulation 92:3014-3024

36. Maxwell LG, Martin LD, Yaster M (1994) Bupivacaine-induced cardiac toxicity in neonates:successful treatment with intravenous phenytoin. Anesthesiology 80:682-686

36. Hubler M, Gabler R, Ehm B et al (2010) Successful resuscitation following opivacaine-induced systemic toxicity in a neonate. Anaesthesia 65:1137-1140
38. Longobardo M, Delpon E, Caballero R et al (1998) Structural determinants of potency and stereoselective block of hKv1.5 channels induced by local anesthetics. Mol Pharmacol 54:162-169
39. Gonzalez T, Arias C, Caballero R et al (2002) Effects of levobupivacaine, ropivacaine and bupivacaine on HERG channels: stereoselective bupivacaine block. Br J Pharmacol 137:1269-1279
40. Valenzuela C, Snyders DJ, Bennett PB et al (1995) Stereoselective block of cardiac sodium channels by bupivacaine in guinea pig ventricular myocytes. Circulation 92:3014-3024
41. Komai H, Lokuta AJ (1999) Interaction of bupivacaine and tetracaine with the sarcoplasmic reticulum Ca2+ release channel of skeletal and cardiac muscles. Anesthesiology 90:835-843
42. Zapata-Sudo G, Trachez MM, Sudo RT et al (2001) Is comparative cardiotoxicity of S() and R(+) bupivacaine related to enantio- mer-selective inhibition of L-type Ca(2+) channels? Anesth Analg 92:496-501
43. Raymond SA, Thalhammer JG, Strichartz GR (1989) Axonal excitability: endogenous and exogenous modulation, in Dimitrijevic Ed Altered sensation and Pain. Recent Achievement in Restorative Neurology, Vol 3, Karger Basel 1990, cited by Raymond SA and Strichartz GR. The long and short of differential block (Editorial). Anesthesiology 70:725-728
44. Vabnick I, Novakovic SD, Levinson SR et al (1996) The clustering of axonal sodium channels during development of the peripheral nervous system. J Neurosci 16:4914- 4922
45. Rasband MN, Trimmer JS (2001) Developmental clustering of ion channels at and near the node of Ranvier. Dev Biol 236:5-16
46. Kohane DS, Sankar WN, Shubina M et al (1998) Sciatic nerve blockade in infant, adolescent, and adult rats: a comparison of ropivacaine with bupivacaine. Anesthesiology 89:1199-1208
47. Greitz D, Hannerz J (1996) A proposed model of cerebrospinal fluid circulation: observations with radionuclide cisternography. AJNR Am J Neuroradiol 17:431-438
48. Wachi A, Kudo S, Sato K (1989) Characteristics of cerebrospinal fluid circulation in infants as detected with MR velocity imaging. Acta Anaesthesiol Scand 33:385-388
49. Booth D, Evans DJ (2004) Anticonvulsants for neonates with seizures. Cochrane Database Syst Rev 4:CD004218
50. de La Coussaye J, Brugada J, Allessie MA (1992) Electrophysiologic and arrhythmogenic-effects of bupivacaine. A study with high-resolution ventricular epicardial mapping in rabbit hearts. Anesthesiology 77:32-41
51. Mazoit JX, Decaux A, Bouaziz H et al (2000) Comparative ventricular electrophysiologic effect of racemic bupivacaine, levobupivacaine, and ropivacaine on the isolated rabbit heart. Anesthesiology 93:784-792
52. Simon L, Kariya N, Edouard A et al (2004) Effect of bupivacaine on the isolated rabbit heart: developmental aspect on ventricular conduction and contractility. Anesthesiology 101:937-944
53. Odoom JA, Sturk A, Dokter PWC et al (1989) The effects of bupivacaine and pipecoloxylidide on platelet function in vitro. Acta Anaesthesiol Scand 33:385-388
54. Hollmann MW, Gross A, Jelacin N et al (2001) Local anesthetic effects on priming and activation of human neutrophils. Anesthesiology 95:113-122
55. Beloeil H, Asehnoune K, Moine P et al (2005) Bupivacaine's action on the carrageenan induced inflammatory response in mice: cytokine production by leukocytes after ex-vivo stimulation. Anesth Analg 100:1081-1086
56. Leduc C, Gentili ME, Estèbe JP et al (2002) Inhibition of peroxydation by local anesthetic in an inflammatory rat model with carrageenan. Anesth Analg 95:992-996
57. Rowbotham MC, Reisner-Keller LA, Fields HL (1991) Both intravenous lidocaine and morphine reduce the pain of postherpetic neuralgia. Neurology 41:1024-1028

58. Marret E, Rolin M, Beaussier M et al (2008) Meta-analysis of intravenous lidocaine and postoperative recovery after abdominal surgery. Br J Surg 95:1331-1338
59. Linchitz RM, Raheb JC (1999) Subcutaneous infusion of lidocaine provides effective pain relief for CRPS patients. Clin J Pain 15:67-72
60. Dadure C, Motais F, Ricard C et al (2005) Con enantiomers on intracellular Ca2+ regulation in murine skeletal muscle fibers. Anesthesiology 102:793-798
61. Popitz-Bergez FA, Leeson S, Strichartz GR et al (1995) Relation between functional deficit and intraneural local anesthetic during peripheral nerve block. A study in the rat sciatic nerve. Anesthesiology 83:583-592
62. Zink W, Missler G, Sinner B et al (2005) Differential effects of bupivacaine and ropivacaine enantiomers on intracellular Ca2+ regulation in murine skeletal muscle fibers. Anesthesiology 102:793-798
63. Nouette-Gaulain K, Sirvent P, Canal-Raffin M et al (2007) Effects of intermittent femoral nerve injections of bupivacaine, levobupivacaine, and ropivacaine on mitochondrial energy metabolism and intracellular calcium homeostasis in rat psoas muscle. Anesthesiology 106:1026-1034
64. Brown DL, Ransom DM, Hall JA et al (1995) Regional anesthesia and local anesthetic induced systemic toxicity: seizure frequency and accompanying cardiovascular changes. Anesth Analg 81:321-328
65. Di Gregorio G, Neal JM, Rosenquist RW et al (2010) Clinical presentation of local anesthetic systemic toxicity: a review of published cases, 1979 to 2009. Reg Anesth Pain Med 35:181-187
66. Weinberg GL (2010) Treatment of local anesthetic systemic toxicity (LAST). Reg Anesth Pain Med 35:188-193
67. Rosenblatt MA, Abel M, Fischer GW et al (2006) Successful use of a 20% lipid emulsion to resuscitate a patient after a presumed bupivacaine-related cardiac arrest. Anesthesiology 105:217-218
68. Litz RJ, Popp M, Stehr SN et al (2009) Successful lipid emulsions. Anesthesiology 110:380-386
69. Ludot H, Tharin JY, Belouadah M et al (2008) Successful resuscitation after ropivacaine and lidocaine-induced ventricular arrhythmia following posterior lumbar plexus block in a child. Anesth Analg 106:1572-1574
70. Mazoit JX, Le Guen R, Beloeil H et al (2009) Binding of long-lasting local anesthetics to lipid emulsions. Anesthesiology 110:380-386
71. Flandin-Bléty C, Barrier G (1995) Accidents following extradural analgesia in children. The results of a retrospective study. Paediatr Anaesth 5:41-46
72. Jamali S, Monin S, Begon C et al (1994) Clonidine in pediatric caudal anesthesia. Anesth Analg 78:663-666
73. Hansen TG, Henneberg SW, Walther Larsen S et al (2004) Caudal bupivacaine supplemented with caudal or intravenous clonidine in children undergoing hypospadias repair: a double-blind study. Br J Anaesth 92:223-227
74. De Negri P, Ivani G, Visconti C et al (2001) How to prolong postoperative analgesia after caudal anaesthesia with ropivacaine in children: S-ketamine versus clonidine. Paediatr Anaesth 11:679-683
75. Braun S, Gaza N, Werdehausen R et al (2010) Ketamine induces apoptosis via the mitochondrial pathway in human lymphocytes and neuronal cells. Br J Anaesth 105:347-354
76. Eisenach JC, Yaksh TL (2003) Epidural ketamine in healthy children – what is the point? Anesth Analg 96:626
77. Lejus C, Surbled M, Schwoerer D et al (2001) Postoperative epidural analgesia with bupivacaine and fentanyl: hourly pain assessment in 348 paediatric cases. Paediatr Anaesth 11:327-332
78. Luz G, Innerhofer I, Bachmann B et al (1996) Bupivacaine plasma concentrations during continuous epidural anesthesia in infants and children. Anesth Analg 82:231-234

Awareness Monitoring in Children

13

Andrew J. Davidson

13.1 Introduction

Several recent studies have demonstrated that children may be at greater risk of awareness than adults [1–6]. The reasons why children are more likely to be aware are unknown. It is difficult to know how to prevent awareness in children without a clear understanding of what is causing it. While there is some evidence that depth-of-anesthesia monitors may decrease the risk of awareness in adults, there is no direct evidence to suggest that they do so in children.

13.2 Definition of Awareness

Before discussing awareness, it is important to provide a working definition. There are several definitions of awareness. The most relevant of these is the explicit recall of events that occurred during anesthesia. Explicit recall is memory which is consciously recalled.

Other definitions include being awake and responsive during anesthesia (with or without any recall of the event). It is also possible that patients may be awake, have no explicit recall, but have implicit memory. Implicit memory is memory which leads to alterations in behavior, but without conscious recollection. Finally, there is some evidence that implicit memory may form without being awake.

A.J. Davidson (✉)
Anesthesia Department, Royal Children's Hospital,
Flemington Road, Parkville, Victoria, Australia
e-mail: andrew.davidson@rch.org.au

M. Astuto (ed.) *Pediatric Anesthesia, Intensive Care and Pain: Standardization in Clinical Practice.* Anesthesia, Intensive Care and Pain in Neonates and Children
DOI: 10.1007/978-88-470-2685-8_13, © Springer-Verlag Italia 2013

13.3   The Incidence of Awareness in Children

In 2007, a survey of pediatric anesthesiologists found that 27% had noted at least one case of pediatric awareness [7]. There are several cohort studies that have been designed to determine the incidence of awareness in children [1–5,8–10]. In 1973, McKie and Thorp reported an incidence of 5% among 202 children aged 7–14 [9]. In contrast, in 1988, two small studies found no cases of awareness [8, 10]. More recently, a larger study in 864 children found an incidence of 0.8% [2]. Later, the same group conducted another study in 500 children [3]. In this study, they adopted an idea originally described by Brice and colleagues [11] where the specificity of the assessment was increased by playing distinct noises to patients during anesthesia. Using this technique, they found an incidence of only 0.2%. In Switzerland, Lopez and colleagues conducted a study in 410 children finding 1.2% to be aware [4], and in The Netherlands, a study in 928 children found an incidence of 0.6% [1]. Lastly, a multicenter study in the United States found an incidence of 0.8% from a cohort of 1,784 children [5]. The data from the most recent five studies were pooled to give a total incidence of 0.7% [6].

There are other cases where awareness in children has been described, such as three case series describing the psychological consequences of awareness, which included at least some adults who would have been children when such awareness had occurred [12–14]. There have also been published case reports [15]; three small studies assessing implicit memory in children found no evidence for explicit memory [16–18] and two studies designed to determine wakefulness noted no explicit recall [19,20].

These studies report a wide range of incidence. High rates in the original study [9] may have been due to outdated anesthesia techniques and, given that awareness is relatively unusual, the smaller studies which found no awareness may not have been sufficiently powerful. Lastly, several studies used only indirect and insensitive methods to detect awareness. The best estimate may be the 0.7% derived from the pooled study [6]. This is higher than the rates usually described in adults.

13.4   Problems in Measuring Awareness

Determining if a reported memory is awareness or if it is a memory of events either before or after surgery is problematic, and this can be more so in children. Similarly, people may report dreams or other false memories. In adult studies, researchers have standardized studies by using an interview similar to that originally described by Brice and colleagues [11]. However, this interview is unsuitable for children as they have less developed memory encoding and consolidation, and less developed memory retrieval strategies [4]. Awareness may be underestimated if questions are open ended and lack context; it may also be overestimated if the questions are suggestive, and as children typically report fragmentary memory rather than detailed memory. Thus, poor interview techniques can result in awareness being either under- or overreported in children.

Children also cannot easily remember when an event occurred (this is known as poor source monitoring) and hence they may more easily attribute a preoperative event as awareness. For example, in one awareness study children were played the sound of a train preoperatively and several children later reported they heard a train during the operation [3].

13.5 Characteristics of Awareness in Children

In adults, awareness is often not volunteered and there may be some delay in reporting [21]. Adults usually report hearing things but they may also report pain or feeling paralysed. In adults, awareness may be associated with tachycardia or hypertension, but these signs are nonspecific and do not always indicate awareness [22]. Awareness in children has some similar characteristics. In children, awareness is often not volunteered to hospital staff, though some children may tell their family. Reporting may also be delayed. Children also describe hearing things, but tend to report more tactile experiences than adults and less pain. The majority of adults are distressed by awareness [23], while it has been suggested that some children may be less distressed by awareness than adults, though for some children the event is without doubt very distressing. In children, memories may be more fragmentary and less rich in detail.

13.6 Causes of Awareness in Children

In adults, awareness is most commonly due to error in anesthetic technique and/or inadvertent light anesthesia [24, 25]. Awareness may also occur in adults when the patient cannot tolerate larger doses of anesthesia (trauma); if signs of light anesthesia are not detectable, such as in cardiopulmonary bypass or with neuromuscular blocking agents; or when agent monitoring is unreliable (bronchoscopy). For some cases the cause is uncertain and may be due to genetic variation in anesthesia requirement.

In children, the causes are not well known. It is logical to expect that some of the risk factors in adults would be applicable to children, such as error and cardiopulmonary bypass. In the pooled pediatric cohort studies, the only identified risk factors were the use of nitrous oxide or the use of a tracheal tube. It is unclear why these were risk factors.

There are several theoretical reasons why awareness may be higher in children. The first is that the report of awareness may not be accurate (as discussed previously). Another possibility is that there may be particular aspects of pediatric anesthesia that increase risk. It has been suggested that the use of induction rooms increases the risk as, when the child is disconnected from the circuit for transfer to the operating room, this may allow the breathing of ambient air, the lightening of anesthesia, and hence increase the risk of awareness [26]. This is unlikely, as induction rooms were not used in some of the studies where high incidences were nonetheless recorded [4, 5].

There are some differences in the pharmacology of the anesthetics used in children that may increase the risk of awareness. Children have a higher minimum alveolar concentration (MAC). In general, MAC peaks in infancy then declines with increasing age [27, 28]. When considering awareness, being "MAC awake" is more relevant than MAC. "MAC awake" is the end-tidal concentration of an anesthetic agent at which 50% of patients appropriately respond to verbal commands [29]. "MAC awake" is also higher in children and declines with age; the ratio of MAC to "MAC awake" remains fairly constant [30–33]. In contrast to "MAC awake", the ratio of the bispectral index (BIS) and entropy to MAC changes with age. The degree to which the electroencephalograph (EEG) is suppressed at 1 MAC is lower in children [34–38], though the relevance of this with regard to awareness is unknown.

As children require more anesthetic, it is possible that awareness is more common simply because anesthesiologists do not give high-enough doses or concentrations, or because they do not wait long enough for the effect-site concentrations to rise. There is no evidence to support this; however, it is interesting to note that in the two Australian studies the incidence of awareness was much lower in the second study where the anesthesiologists knew that awareness was being assessed.

13.7 Consequences of Awareness in Children

In adults, the psychological consequences of awareness vary from bored indifference to post-traumatic stress disorder (PTSD). In adult prospective studies, the incidence of severe psychological disturbance such as PTSD is between 0% and 44% [12–14, 39–41]. It is important to note that severe disturbance may only be apparent some time after the event, and significant psychological consequences are more likely when the memory is detailed or if the patient felt as if they were paralysed [42].

There are only limited data on the consequences of awareness in children. As mentioned previously, several studies that examined psychological outcomes after awareness included adults that would have had their awareness experience as children. Several had PTSD or other evidence of severe psychological disturbance [12–14]. In contrast, in the recent cohort studies, there was very little if any evidence of psychological consequences [2, 43, 44]. While some children certainly can develop PTSD after awareness, the incidence may be lower than in adults. The reasons for this are unclear, but may be due to the finding that fewer aware children felt paralysed.

13.8 Monitoring for Awareness

There are several ways to monitor for awareness. The simplest is to watch for signs of light anesthesia such as movement, coughing, tachycardia, and hypertension; however, these are all nonspecific signs. Another way is to ensure that an adequate dose of anesthesia is delivered through end-tidal agent monitoring. In adults, there is evidence that following a strict protocol that aims for minimum end-tidal concentrations of volatile anesthetics may reduce the incidence of awareness, though it is unclear if this is more or less effective than BIS monitoring [45, 46].

Heart rate variability, skin conductance, pupil size and reactivity [47, 48], and esophageal tone have all been used to measure anesthesia depth with limited success or use. These techniques have not been widely assessed in children. The isolated forearm technique is very occasionally used and mostly for research [20]. In this technique, a tourniquet is applied to the patient's upper arm and is inflated above systolic blood pressure before neuromuscular blocking agents are administered. Movement of the arm, either spontaneously or in response to commands, such as the patient being repeatedly asked to squeeze their fingers, indicate wakefulness.

It has long been known that the EEG changes with different doses of anesthetic. Increasing concentrations of anesthetics such as propofol and isoflurane initially increase the power of the EEG and produce a shift from α to faster β frequencies. With further increases in concentration, the total power falls and there is a shift to the much slower δ frequencies. Very high concentrations result in burst suppression, high-voltage activity alternating with isoelectric quiescence which is commonly observed at deep levels of general anesthesia. For ketamine, halothane, nitrous oxide, xenon, or high doses of opioids, the relative effects on the EEG are less predictable. The auditory evoked potential (AEP) is the change in the EEG produced by an auditory stimulus; it can also be used to measure anesthesia depth.

13.9 Depth-of-Anesthesia Monitors

Faster EEG analysis has allowed the development of several devices that use various mathematical properties of the passive EEG to measure anesthesia depth. The EEG signal is collected from 3–4 scalp electrodes. The signal is digitized, filtered for artifact, and then analyzed in a variety of different ways depending on the monitor. An entropy monitor calculates Shannon entropy and a BIS monitor computes the ratio of power in fast and slow frequencies and the bispectral power. Many of the monitors use several different analyses combined into a single algorithm. Separate analysis is often needed to specifically detect burst suppression.

In adults, the commercially available depth-of-anesthesia monitors have all been shown to be responsive to changes in the concentration of propofol or volatile anesthetics, such as isoflurane; however, the correlation is not perfect. Monitors also have some capacity to differentiate between the awake and the unconscious state; however, once again this is not perfect and there is inevitably some overlap in output numbers between awake and unconscious states. Generally speaking, the lower the number, the greater the probability that the patient is unconscious. There are very few studies that have directly compared monitors. There is mixed evidence that depth-of-anesthesia monitors reduce the incidence of awareness in high-risk adult patients [45,46,49].

There are recognized, specific limitations to depth-of-anesthesia monitors. There is some evidence that neuromuscular blockade may influence the monitors. At deep levels of anesthesia, it seems that the blockade has no effect [50]. However, it is possible that neuromuscular blocking agents may lower the output number in very lightly anesthetized or completely awake patients [51]. There is also some evidence that the monitors are not as effective in predicting anesthesia depth with agents such as ketamine, xenon, nitrous oxide, high doses of opioids, or halothane [52–54]. It has also been shown that the BIS initially falls as sevoflurane concentrations increase, but for concentrations greater than 3% the BIS will paradoxically increase with further increases in sevoflurane concentrations [55,56]. Lastly, many children undergoing anesthesia have a learning or behavioral disability. There is some evidence that the performance of depth-of-anesthesia monitors may be different in this group of patients [57].

13.10 Depth-of-Anesthesia Monitors in Children

The awake EEG changes with age. When anesthetized, the power of the EEG is also much lower in infants less than 6 months old when compared to the EEG of older children [58, 59]. Because the EEG changes with age, depth-of-anesthesia monitors need careful study in children. In general, the performance of monitors in older children is similar to the performance witnessed in adults. In infants, however, monitor performance is very different.

The BIS is the most widely studied depth-of-anesthesia monitor. In older children there is a correlation between the BIS and sevoflurane or isoflurane concentrations [35,60–66]. There is less evidence for correlations between the BIS and propofol concentrations [36,67–70]. When looking at the capacity to differentiate the awake versus the unconscious state, the performance of the BIS as a measure of consciousness is worse in younger children [58]. Although there are very few studies, entropy seems to perform similarly to BIS in children [34, 62,71,72].

There are several studies evaluating the Narcotrend monitor (MonitorTechnik, Bad Bramstedt, Germany) in children. These found a good differentiation between awake and unconscious states and also evidence for a correlation between sevoflurane or desflurane concentrations and the Narcotrend index [73–76]. Monitor performance was not as effective with propofol [77]. There are very few studies investigating the AEP in children during anesthesia. In general, AEP monitors do not perform as well as passive EEG monitors [78,79]. There are also a few studies that have investigated the cerebral state index (CSI) monitor in children; the little data available suggest that the CSI monitor may also be able to measure anesthesia depth in children [80].

13.11 Depth-of-Anesthesia Monitoring and Awareness in Children

There are no studies which specifically test if depth-of-anesthesia monitors decrease awareness in children. Any evidence for or against their use is currently indirect. In older children, the monitors have performance characteristics similar to those described in adults. Thus, if it is accepted that depth-of-anesthesia monitors may reduce awareness in high-risk adults, then it might be expected that they would reduce awareness in high-risk children also. However, this may not be true if the mechanism or the causes of awareness differ in children. As mentioned previously, awareness certainly occurs in children but in most situations it has different characteristics to those seen in adults. Thus, until there are studies specifically investigating the use of depth-of-anesthesia monitors and awareness in children, no firm recommendations can be made. The greatest theoretical benefit is to be found in older children, where the risks of awareness are due to the same mechanisms described in adults, such as trauma. A case could also be made for their use in total intravenous anesthesia (TIVA), because TIVA algorithms are still poorly developed in children.

It is not possible to comment on which monitor would theoretically be best to reduce awareness in children because there are insufficient data comparing their performance in children.

13.12 Use of Depth-of-Anesthesia Monitors outside the Operating Room

Depth-of-anesthesia monitors have also been used to guide sedation in the intensive care unit and in the emergency department. There is only mixed evidence for their effectiveness in adults and very little data about their use in these settings in children [81–83].

13.13 Monitoring for Awareness in Very Young Children

Several studies have found that depth-of-anesthesia monitors perform poorly in infants. Infants have pre-awakening BIS or entropy values lower than older children [34, 60, 71, 84]. Some studies have found it difficult to titrate anesthesia to BIS in infants [85]. This is consistent with a poorer correlation between output numbers and the concentration of the anesthetic agent [34, 71]. The reasons for the poor performance may be due to fundamental differences in the EEG during anesthesia in this age group [58, 86].

Developing a monitor for awareness in infants is difficult as the end points of anesthesia are difficult to define and measure. There is good evidence that infants need effective analgesia and benefit from a reduction in stress, but we have little data on how much anesthetic or analgesic is needed to optimally achieve this. While most people now agree that infants are conscious beings, it is difficult to measure exactly when an infant is awake or unconscious. This makes it difficult to calibrate depth-of-anesthesia monitors or determine the concentration of anesthetic needed for unconsciousness. It is also impossible to measure memory and indeed neonates have no explicit recall. Our means of monitoring awareness in this age group are imprecise and indirect and simply applying the adult paradigms of anesthesia may not be appropriate [87].

References

1. Blusse van Oud-Alblas HJ, van Dijk M, Liu C et al (2009) Intraoperative awareness during pediatric anesthesia. Br J Anaesth 102(1):104-110
2. Davidson AJ, Huang GH, Czarnecki C et al (2005) Awareness during anesthesia in children: a prospective cohort study. Anesth Analg 100(3):653-661, table of contents
3. Davidson AJ, Sheppard SJ, Engwerda AL et al (2008) Detecting awareness in children by using an auditory intervention. Anesthesiology 109(4):619-624
4. Lopez U, Habre W, Laurencon M et al (2007) Intra-operative awareness in children: the value of an interview adapted to their cognitive abilities. Anesthesia 62(8):778-89
5. Malviya S, Galinkin JL, Bannister CF et al (2009) The incidence of intraoperative awareness in children: childhood awareness and recall evaluation. Anesth Analg 109(5):1421-1427
6. Davidson AJ, Smith KR, Blusse van Oud-Alblas HJ et al (2011) Awareness in children: a secondary analysis of five cohort studies. Anesthesia 66(6):446-454
7. Engelhardt T, Petroz GC, McCheyne A et al (2007) Awareness during pediatric anesthesia: what is the position of European pediatric anesthesiologists? Paediatr Anaesth 17(11):1066-1070
8. Hobbs AJ, Bush GH, Downham DY (1988) Peri-operative dreaming and awareness in children. Anesthesia 43(7):560-562
9. McKie BD, Thorp EA (1973) Awareness and dreaming during anesthesia in a pediatric hospital. Anaesth Intensive Care 1(5):407-414
10. O'Sullivan EP, Childs D, Bush GH (1988) Peri-operative dreaming in pediatric patients who receive suxamethonium. Anesthesia 43(2):104-106
11. Brice DD, Hetherington RR, Utting JE (1970) A simple study of awareness and dreaming during anesthesia. Br J Anaesth 42(6):535-542
12. Samuelsson P, Brudin L, Sandin RH (2007) Late psychological symptoms after awareness among consecutively included surgical patients. Anesthesiology 106(1):26-32
13. Schwender D, Kunze-Kronawitter H, Dietrich P et al (1998) Conscious awareness during general anesthesia: patients' perceptions, emotions, cognition and reactions. Br J Anaesth 80(2):133-139
14. Osterman JE, van der Kolk BA (1998) Awareness during anesthesia and posttraumatic stress disorder. Gen Hosp Psychiatry 20(5):274-281

15. Blusse Vano-Ahj, Bosenberg AT, Tibboel D (2008) Awareness in children: another two cases. Paediatr Anaesth

16. Bonke B, Van Dam ME, Van Kleff JW et al (1992) Implicit memory tested in children during inhalation anesthesia. Anesthesia 47(9):747-749

17. Kalff AC, Bonke B, Wolters G et al (1995) Implicit memory for stimuli presented during inhalation anesthesia in children. Psychol Rep 77(2):371-375

18. Rich JB, Yaster M, Brandt J (1999) Anterograde and retrograde memory in children anesthetized with propofol. J Clin Exp Neuropsychol 21(4):535-546

19. Byers GF, Muir JG (1997) Detecting wakefulness in anaesthetised children. Can J Anaesth 44(5 Pt 1):486-488

20. Andrade J, Deeprose C, Barker I (2008) Awareness and memory function during pediatric anesthesia. Br J Anaesth 100(3):389-396

21. Sandin RH, Enlund G, Samuelsson P et al (2000) Awareness during anesthesia: a prospective case study. Lancet 355(9205):707-711

22. Moerman N, Bonke B, Oosting J (1993) Awareness and recall during general anesthesia. Facts and feelings. Anesthesiology 79(3):454-464

23. Myles PS, Williams DL, Hendrata M et al (2000) Patient satisfaction after anesthesia and surgery: results of a prospective survey of 10,811 patients. Br J Anaesth 84(1):6-10

24. Domino KB, Posner KL, Caplan RA et al (1999) Awareness during anesthesia: a closed claims analysis. Anesthesiology 90(4):1053-1061

25. Errando CL, Sigl JC, Robles M et al (2008) Awareness with recall during general anesthesia: a prospective observational evaluation of 4001 patients. Br J Anaesth

26. Davis PJ (2005) Goldilocks: the pediatric anesthesiologist's dilemma. Anesthesia & Analgesia 100(3):650-652

27. Lerman J, Sikich N, Kleinman S et al (1994) The pharmacology of sevoflurane in infants and children. Anesthesiology 80(4):814-824

28. Brosnan RJ, Pypendop BH, Barter LS et al (2006) Pharmacokinetics of inhaled anesthetics in green iguanas (Iguana iguana) Am J Vet Res 67(10):1670-1674

29. Eger EI (2001) 2nd Age, minimum alveolar anesthetic concentration, and minimum alveolar anesthetic concentration-awake. Anesth Analg 93(4):947-953

30. Inomata S, Kihara S, Miyabe M et al (2002) The hypnotic and analgesic effects of oral clonidine during sevoflurane anesthesia in children: a dose-response study. Anesth Analg 94(6):1479-1483

31. Mapleson WW (1996) Effect of age on MAC in humans: a meta-analysis. Br J Anaesth 76(2):179-185

32. Kihara S, Inomata S, Yaguchi Y et al (2000) The awakening concentration of sevoflurane in children. Anesth Analg 91(2):305-308

33. Katoh T, Suguro Y, Ikeda T et al (1993) Influence of age on awakening concentrations of sevoflurane and isoflurane. Anesth Analg 76(2):348-352

34. Davidson AJ, Huang GH, Rebmann CS et al (2005) Performance of entropy and Bispectral Index as measures of anesthesia effect in children of different ages. Br J Anaesth 95(5):674-679

35. Wodey E, Tirel O, Bansard JY et al (2005) Impact of age on both BIS values and EEG bispectrum during anesthesia with sevoflurane in children. British Journal of Anesthesia 94(6):810-820

36. Tirel O, Wodey E, Harris R et al (2008) Variation of bispectral index under TIVA with propofol in a pediatric population. Br J Anaesth 100(1):82-87

37. Tirel O, Wodey E, Harris R et al (2006) The impact of age on bispectral index values and EEG bispectrum during anesthesia with desflurane and halothane in children. Br J Anaesth 96(4):480-485

38. Tsuruta S, Satsumae T, Mizutani T et al (2011) Minimum alveolar concentrations of sevoflurane for maintaining bispectral index below 50 in children. Paediatr Anaesth 221(11):1124-1127

39. Wennervirta J, Ranta SO, Hynynen M (2002) Awareness and recall in outpatient anesthesia. Anesth Analg 95(1):72-77, table of contents

40. Lennmarken C, Bildfors K, Enlund G et al (2002) Victims of awareness. Acta Anaesthesiol Scand 46(3):229-231

41. Ranta SO, Laurila R, Saario J et al (1998) Awareness with recall during general anesthesia: incidence and risk factors. Anesth Analg 86(5):1084-1089

42. Leslie K, Chan MT, Myles PS et al (2010) Posttraumatic stress disorder in aware patients from the B-aware trial. Anesth Analg 110(3):823-828

43. Phelan L, Stargatt R, Davidson AJ (2009) Long-term posttraumatic effects of intraoperative awareness in children. Paediatr Anaesth 19(12):1152-1156

44. Lopez U, Habre W, Van der Linden M et al (2008) Intra-operative awareness in children and post-traumatic stress disorder. Anesthesia 63(5):474-481

45. Avidan MS, Zhang L, Burnside BA et al (2008) Anesthesia awareness and the bispectral index. N Engl J Med 358(11):1097-1108

46. Avidan MS, Jacobsohn E, Glick D et al (20011) Prevention of intraoperative awareness in a high-risk surgical population. N Engl J Med 365(7):591-600

47. Bourgeois E, Sabourdin N, Louvet N et al (2012) Minimal alveolar concentration of sevoflurane inhibiting the reflex pupillary dilatation after noxious stimulation in children and young adults. Br J Anaesth 108(4):648-654

48. Constant I, Nghe MC, Boudet L et al (2006) Reflex pupillary dilatation in response to skin incision and alfentanil in children anaesthetized with sevoflurane: a more sensitive measure of noxious stimulation than the commonly used variables. Br J Anaesth 96(5):614-619

49. Myles PS, Leslie K, McNeil J et al (2004) Bispectral index monitoring to prevent awareness during anesthesia: the B-Aware randomised controlled trial. Lancet 363(9423):1757-1763

50. Weber F, Kriek N, Blusse van Oud-Alblas HJ (2010) The effects of mivacurium-induced neuromuscular block on Bispectral Index and Cerebral State Index in children under propofol anesthesia - a prospective randomized clinical trial. Paediatr Anaesth 20(8):697-703

51. Messner M, Beese U, Romstock J et al (2003) The bispectral index declines during neuromuscular block in fully awake persons. Anesth Analg 97(2):488-491 table of contents

52. Davidson AJ, Czarnecki C (2004) The Bispectral Index in children: comparing isoflurane and halothane. Br J Anaesth 92(1):14-17

53. Davidson A (2004) The correlation between bispectral index and airway reflexes with sevoflurane and halothane anesthesia. Paediatr Anaesth 14(3):241-246

54. Edwards JJ, Soto RG, Bedford RF (2005) Bispectral Index values are higher during halothane vs. sevoflurane anesthesia in children, but not in infants. Acta Anaesthesiol Scand 49(8):1084-1087

55. Constant I, Leport Y, Richard P et al (2004) Agitation and changes of Bispectral Index and electroencephalographic-derived variables during sevoflurane induction in children: clonidine premedication reduces agitation compared with midazolam. Br J Anaesth 92(4):504-511

56. Kim HS, Oh AY, Kim CS et al (2005) Correlation of bispectral index with end-tidal sevoflurane concentration and age in infants and children. Br J Anaesth 95(3):362-366

57. Valkenburg AJ, de Leeuw TG, Tibboel D et al (2009) Lower bispectral index values in children who are intellectually disabled. Anesth Analg 109(5):1428-1433

58. Davidson AJ, Sale SM, Wong C et al (2008) The electroencephalograph during anesthesia and emergence in infants and children. Paediatr Anaesth 18(1):60-70

59. McKeever S, Johnston L, Davidson AJ (2012) An observational study exploring amplitude-integrated electroencephalogram and spectral edge frequency during pediatric anesthesia. Anaesth Intensive Care 40(2):275-284

60. Davidson AJ, McCann ME, Devavaram P et al (2001) The differences in the bispectral index between infants and children during emergence from anesthesia after circumcision surgery. Anesth Analg 93(2):326-330

61. Denman WT, Swanson EL, Rosow D, et al (2000) Pediatric evaluation of the bispectral index (BIS) monitor and correlation of BIS with end-tidal sevoflurane concentration in infants and children. Anesth Analg 90(4):872-877

62. Davidson AJ, Kim MJ, Sangolt GK (2004) Entropy and bispectral index during anesthesia in children. Anesthesia & Intensive Care 32(4):485-493

63. McCann ME, Bacsik J, Davidson A et al (2002) The correlation of bispectral index with endtidal sevoflurane concentration and haemodynamic parameters in preschoolers. Paediatr Anaesth 12(6):519-525

64. Brosius KK, Bannister CF et al (2002) Oral midazolam premedication in preadolescents and adolescents. Anesth Analg 94(1):31-36

65. Brosius KK, Bannister CF (2001) Effect of oral midazolam premedication on the awakening concentration of sevoflurane, recovery times and bispectral index in children. Paediatr Anaesth 11(5):585-590

66. Whyte SD, Booker PD (2004) Bispectral index during isoflurane anesthesia in pediatric patients. Anesth Analg 98(6):1644-1649

67. Park HJ, Kim YL, Kim CS et al (2007) Changes of bispectral index during recovery from general anesthesia with 2% propofol and remifentanil in children. Paediatr Anaesth 17(4):353-357

68. Munoz HR, Cortinez LI, Ibacache ME et al (2006) Effect site concentrations of propofol producing hypnosis in children and adults: comparison using the bispectral index. Acta Anaesthesiol Scand 50(7):882-887

69. Degoute CS, Macabeo C, Dubreuil C et al (2001) EEG bispectral index and hypnotic component of anesthesia induced by sevoflurane: comparison between children and adults. Br J Anaesth 86(2):209-212

70. Rigouzzo A, Girault L, Louvet N et al (2008) The relationship between bispectral index and propofol during target-controlled infusion anesthesia: a comparative study between children and young adults. Anesth Analg 106(4):1109-1116, table of contents

71. Klockars JG, Hiller A, Ranta S et al (2006) Spectral entropy as a measure of hypnosis in children. Anesthesiology 104(4):708-717

72. Klockars JG, Hiller A, Munte S et al (2012) Spectral entropy as a measure of hypnosis and hypnotic drug effect of total intravenous anesthesia in children during slow induction and maintenance. Anesthesiology 116(2):340-351

73. Weber F, Hollnberger H, Gruber M et al (2004) Narcotrend depth of anesthesia monitoring in infants and children. Can J Anaesth 51(8):855-856

74. Weber F, Gruber M, Taeger K (2005) The correlation of the Narcotrend Index and classical electroencephalographic parameters with endtidal desflurane concentrations and hemodynamic parameters in different age groups. Paediatr Anaesth 15(5):378-384

75. Weber F, Hollnberger H, Gruber M et al (2005) The correlation of the Narcotrend Index with endtidal sevoflurane concentrations and hemodynamic parameters in children. Paediatr Anaesth 15(9):727-732

76. Wallenborn J, Kluba K, Olthoff D (2007) Comparative evaluation of Bispectral Index and Narcotrend Index in children below 5 years of age. Paediatr Anaesth 17(2):140-147

77. Munte S, Klockars J, van Gils M et al (2009) The Narcotrend index indicates age-related changes during propofol induction in children. Anesth Analg 109(1):53-59

78. Weber F, Bein T, Hobbhahn J et al (2004) Evaluation of the Alaris Auditory Evoked Potential Index as an indicator of anesthetic depth in preschool children during induction of anesthesia with sevoflurane and remifentanil. Anesthesiology 101(2):294-298

79. Ironfield CM, Davidson AJ (2007) AEP-monitor/2 derived, composite auditory evoked potential index (AAI-1.6) and bispectral index as predictors of sevoflurane concentration in children. Paediatr Anaesth 17(5):452-459

80. Disma N, Lauretta D, Palermo F, et al (2007) Level of sedation evaluation with Cerebral State Index and A-Line Arx in children undergoing diagnostic procedures. Paediatr Anaesth 17(5):445-451

81. McKeever S, Johnston L, Davidson A (2012) A review of the utility of EEG depth of anesthesia monitors in the pediatric intensive care environment. Intensive Crit Care Nurs 2012
82. Minardi C, Sahillioglu E, Astuto M, Colombo M, Ingelmo PM (2012) Sedation and analgesia in pediatric intensive care. Curr Drug Targets 13(7):936-943
83. Sammartino M, Volpe B, Sbaraglia F et al (2010) Capnography and the bispectral index-their role in pediatric sedation: a brief review. Int J Pediatr 2010:828347
84. Kawaraguchi Y, Fukumitsu K, Kinouchi K et al (2003) [Bispectral index (BIS) in infants anesthetized with sevoflurane in nitrous oxide and oxygen]. Masui 52(4):389-393
85. Bannister CF, Brosius KK, Sigl JC et al (2001) The effect of bispectral index monitoring on anesthetic use and recovery in children anesthetized with sevoflurane in nitrous oxide. Anesth Analg 92(4):877-881
86. Hayashi K, Shigemi K, Sawa T (2012) Neonatal electroencephalography shows low sensitivity to anesthesia. Neurosci Lett 517(2):87-91
87. Davidson AJ (2012) Neurotoxicity and the need for anesthesia in the newborn: does the emperor have no clothes? Anesthesiology 116(3):507-509

Single-Lung Ventilation in Children: Techniques, Monitoring, and Side Effects

14

Nicola Disma, Leila Mameli, Alessio Pini-Prato,
Girolamo Mattioli and Giovanni Montobbio

14.1 Introduction

Thoracoscopy is increasingly being used for thoracic surgery in both adults and children. Improvements in technology and surgical skills are the main reasons for the dramatic increase in patients being referred for thoracoscopic surgery. As the age and weight of the patients being referred for surgery are declining, newborns and infants are frequently scheduled for thoracoscopic surgery. Deflation of the lung at the surgical site is extremely useful for adequate surgical exposure, especially in the case of pulmonary resection [1].

From an anesthesia point of view, the main obstacle is the performance of reliable single-lung ventilation (SLV) with deflation and immobility of the lung at the surgical site. Double-lumen endobronchial tubes, Univent tubes (Fuji Systems, Tokyo, Japan), and bronchial intubation are some of the techniques described for SLV [2–3]. Alternatively, conventional double-lung ventilation facilitates the collapse of the lung at the surgical site by insufflation of the CO_2 used for the thoracoscopic procedure [4]. These strategies, especially bronchial intubation and double-lung ventilation, cannot be considered as completely satisfactory and should be seen as surrogates of SLV, as described for adult patients. The commercial introduction of the Arndt 5 French (Fr) pediatric endobronchial blocker (COOK MEDICAL Inc., Bloomington, Illinois, USA) for SLV has proved to be a reliable option for SLV, even in children and small infants. The rest of this chapter describes the physiology of SLV in children, the pros and cons of the different devices used in SLV, and the currently available SLV techniques.

N. Disma (✉)
Department of Anesthesia, IRCCS Gaslini Children's Hospital
Genoa, Italy
e-mail: nicoladisma@tin.it

M. Astuto (ed.) *Pediatric Anesthesia, Intensive Care and Pain: Standardization
in Clinical Practice*. Anesthesia, Intensive Care and Pain in Neonates and Children
DOI: 10.1007/978-88-470-2685-8_14, © Springer-Verlag Italia 2013

14.2   Physiology of Single-Lung Ventilation

Ventilation is normally distributed preferentially toward the dependent regions of the lung, with a gradient of increasing ventilation from the nondependent (up) to the dependent lung segments (down). Because of gravitational forces, perfusion normally follows a similar distribution, with increased blood flow toward the dependent lung segments. Therefore, ventilation and perfusion are normally well balanced. During thoracic surgery, several factors interact to affect the ventilation/perfusion (V/Q) balance.

Compression of the dependent lung in the lateral decubitus position and SLV with collapse of the operative lung are both responsible for atelectasis. Hypoxic pulmonary vasoconstriction acts to divert blood flow away from underventilated lung regions, thereby minimizing any V/Q imbalance. However, the overall effect of the lateral decubitus position on the V/Q balance is different in infants compared to older children and adults.

In infants with unilateral lung disease, oxygenation is improved with the healthy lung "up". This physiological phenomenon differs significantly between adults and infants. The main reasons for this difference are the soft and easily compressed thoracic cage and a functional residual capacity closer to the residual volume, which make airway closure likely to occur in the dependent lung even during tidal breathing. Finally, the increased oxygen requirement and the small functional residual capacity predispose children to hypoxemia. All of these factors must be taken into account every time a child undergoes SLV for thoracic surgery.

14.3   Single-Lung Ventilation Techniques

14.3.1 Selective Endobronchial Intubation

This technique is performed by advancing the tracheal tube into one of the mainstem bronchi until breath sounds on the operative side disappear. This is a simple technique that does not require special equipment other than a fiberoptic scope. The main disadvantages are the inability to completely collapse and suction the operative lung, and the incomplete protection of the healthy lung from purulent material or blood originating from the operative side. Moreover, hypoxemia may occur due to obstruction of the upper lobe bronchus, especially when the short right mainstem bronchus is intubated.

14.3.2 Univent Tube

The Univent tube (Fuji Systems, Tokyo, Japan) is a tracheal tube with a second small lumen containing a bronchial blocker (BB). This second lumen can be advanced into the bronchus to be blocked under direct visualization. The BB is firmly attached to the tracheal tube to avoid accidental displacement and a small internal lumen allows lung deflation. Common problems encountered with this device are difficulty in ventilating patients because of the large diameter of the second lumen containing the blocker and the risk of mucosal damage caused by the cuff of the blocker.

14.3.3 Double-Lumen Tubes

Double-lumen tubes (DLTs) are designed as two tubes of unequal length molded together. The shorter tube ends in the trachea and the longer tube in the bronchus. Each lumen has a cuff. The tracheal cuff allows positive ventilation. The bronchial cuff allows separate lung ventilation and protection of each lung from any purulent blood coming from the opposite lung.

Inserting a DLT consists of inserting the tip of the tube through the vocal cords, withdrawing the stylet, rotating the tube 90° to the appropriate side, and then advancing the tip of the tube into the main bronchus. Fiberoptic bronchoscopy is used to confirm tube placement with the bronchial cuff into the main bronchus.

DLTs can be considered the gold standard for SLV. They allow the independent suction and ventilation of each lung and protect both lungs from contamination. Left-sided tubes are preferred to right-sided ones, as they are easier to insert and as right-sided tubes pose a significant risk of right upper lobe obstruction. The main limitation of DLTs is size, as the smallest commercially available size is suitable for teenagers but not younger patients. Therefore, small children cannot benefit from this technique.

14.3.4 The Arndt Bronchial Blocker

We recently published a pediatric case series involving the use of the Arndt BB [5]. The Arndt BB has been designed as a 5 Fr catheter with a distal spherical low-pressure balloon, and a lumen with an inner removable string that exits from the distal end of the catheter. The string can be looped over the fiberoptic scope with the aim of guiding the catheter into the bronchus that is to be blocked. In our study, following removal of the string, the lumen was used for gradual lung collapse at the beginning of thoracoscopy, and for oxygen delivery or aspiration of secretions during surgery. A multiport air adapter is provided with the Arndt BB and this was used to pass the fiberoptic scope and the BB through their respective ports into the tracheal tube (Fig. 14.1). The multiport was connected to the ventilation circuit to manually or mechanically ventilate the patient during the Arndt maneuver. The steps needed for the correct placement of the BB are described in Table 14.1.

The BB is positioned with the patient under general anesthesia. During the procedure, the patient can be ventilated mechanically or manually with 100% oxygen to minimize the risk of hypoxemia. An uncuffed tracheal tube as large as can be tolerated by the patient has to be inserted, with the aim of maximizing

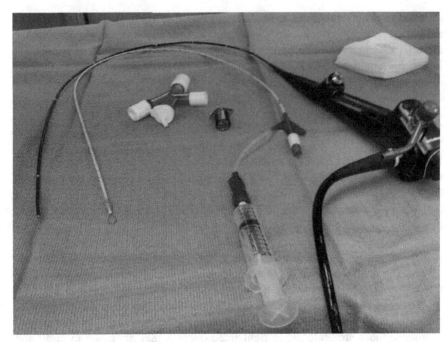

Fig. 14.1 Arndt 5 Fr bronchial blocker, multiport air adapter, and 2.7 mm fiberscope

Table 14.1 Steps for correct bronchial blocker (BB) positioning

1. The BB and scope are introduced through the ports.
2. The scope is passed into the loop of the BB.
3. The scope is advanced into the desired bronchus.
4. Correct identification of the bronchus to be blocked is made.
5. The BB is advanced over the tip of the scope.
6. The scope is pulled back until the carina is visible through the scope.
7. The BB is moved back to the main bronchus to be blocked.
8. The balloon is inflated under direct visualization (within a volume of air up to 2 mL).
9. Placement of the inflated balloon in the bronchus is confirmed by direct visualization and auscultation of lung separation.
10. The BB port is tightened following the removal of the fiberoptic scope to allow correct ventilation.

the space available for the maneuver with the fiberscope and BB inside the tube (Table 14.1).

In our study, we were able to achieve SLV in all patients of the case series. Placement required approximately 10–25 min. SLV was tolerated in all patients; a continuous positive flow of oxygen with a measured pressure of 10–15 cm H_2O was delivered into the blocked lung through the lumen of the Arndt BB in patients with reduced intraoperative tolerance of SLV. The main adverse event was

BB displacement, especially when patients were turned onto their side. For this reason, the BB can be safely placed in patients already turned onto their side for surgery in such cases. Except for the reported displacement, there were no reported complications from BB placement and SLV was successful even in very young patients.

14.4 Discussion

SLV is a helpful technique for thoracic surgery. It can be mandatory in the case of thoracoscopy, when the need for a good surgical view and enough space to maneuver have a significant impact on the final outcome. Different devices and techniques have been presented in this chapter, such as choosing the correct tube size (Table 14.2), but the two most reliable devices are the Arndt BB and the DLT. Considering the age of pediatric patients, the only commercially available option is the Arndt BB, as the smallest size of the DLT is only suitable for adolescents. We published a first study using a 5 Fr BB in children undergoing thoracoscopic surgery. The device has been shown to be a reliable method to achieve SLV, being extremely helpful for both thoracoscopy and video-assisted thoracic surgery in selected cases or for major lung surgery and surgery involving the mediastinal structures of relatively young patients, and several case series have been published [5–6]. Our experience suggests that BB should be used in young patients where the DLT cannot be used.

First, the main benefit of using the Arndt BB is that it can be passed through a standard tracheal tube; this should be easier to learn and master, especially in a large pediatric hospital where thoracic surgery is relatively frequent. All the anesthesiologists involved were interested in thoracic anesthesia and had specific expertise in airway management and pediatric bronchoscopy. For this reason, achieving proficiency in positioning a BB was relatively rapid and displacements were the only reported adverse events.

Table 14.2 Tube size selection for single-lung ventilation in infants, children, and teenagers

Age (years)	ETT (ID in mm)	BB (Fr)	Univent (ID in mm)	DLT (Fr)
0.5–1	3.5–4.0	5	–	–
1–2	4.0–4.5	5	–	–
2–4	4.5–5.0	5	–	–
4–6	5.0–5.5	5	–	–
6–8	5.5–6.5	5	3.5	24
8–10	6.0–6.5	5	3.5	26
10–12	6.5–7.0	5–7	4.5	26–28
12–14	7.0–7.5	5–7	4.5	32

BB bronchial blocker, *DLT* double-lumen tube, *ETT* endotracheal tube, *Fr* French size (medical tubing unit of measurement), *ID* inner diameter

A comparison between the BB and a different device, such as the DLT, has already been published in adults [7–8]. The authors concluded that each device provides advantages, depending on each specific case and that a "best" device does not exist. In particular, for absolute lung separation, the use of the DLT has been shown to be the best choice. On the other hand, the BB represents a better choice for patients with difficult airways or for selective lobar ventilation. A similar comparison is not feasible in children because of the lack of commercially available pediatric devices.

Second, the size of the tracheal tube and consequently the age and weight of the patient can be considered a limitation for performing lung separation with a BB. The smallest tracheal tube used in the present series had a 5.5 mm internal diameter (ID) and the blocker was positioned under direct visualization using a 2.8 mm fiberoptic scope. If a smaller tracheal tube were to be used, then a 2 mm fiberoptic scope would be required for the procedure. A recently published article [9] described the insertion of a 5 Fr BB outside the tracheal tube in an infant aged less than 1 year. Placing a BB outside the tracheal tube is an alternative option which can be applied in small children, but it is far from being routine clinical practice.

In our clinical practice, the tracheal tube connector is substituted with a larger one, outside the extremity of the tube. The connector between the tracheal tube and the breathing circuit is the narrowest point and the space to maneuver the scope and the BB can be limited, especially with the smaller tubes (5.5 mm ID or smaller). For this reason, the connector is routinely changed with a larger one, to be placed outside the tracheal tube and to increase the space to maneuver. A limitation of the technique is the risk of hypoxemia during the insertion of the BB and, intraoperatively, during SLV. We used mechanical or manual ventilation when positioning the BB, and all the patients were deeply anesthetized and immobilized. This was to minimize the risk of hypoxemia, even in the case of air leaking through the multiport. Once the BB was positioned and thoracoscopy started with the operative lung collapsed, a continuous positive airway pressure (CPAP) with a fresh flow of 1–2 L/min O_2 can be established and measured at a pressure of 10–15 cm H_2O, until the end of surgery and lung re-expansion. CPAP works by improving oxygenation. The ventilator can be set up using pressure-controlled ventilation to minimize the peak inspiratory pressure. Once SLV is started, the peak inspiratory pressure is adjusted to reduce the tidal volume to one-third of that used during double-lung ventilation. The fraction of inspired O2 and the respiratory rate are then adjusted to avoid hypoxemia and hypercarbia [3–4].

14.5 Conclusions

The main difficulty for the correct positioning of a BB is the acquisition of adequate skills in pediatric bronchoscopy and pediatric thoracic anesthesia. The identification of the correct bronchus to be blocked, viewing the upper lobe bronchus on the right or the upper and lower lobar bronchi on the left, knowledge of the devices (fiberoptic scope and BB), and rapid execution of the maneuvers are mandatory for all anesthesiologists involved in pediatric thoracoscopic surgery. The results from our wide-ranging experience in thoracic surgery shows that the Arndt 5 Fr BB is a consistent, reliable, and safe method for SLV in children undergoing thoracoscopic surgery; it can also be used in those cases where DLT ventilation is not suitable because of the young age and low weight of the patient.

References

1. Hammer GB, Fitzmaurice BG, Brodsky JB (1999) Methods for single-lung ventilation in pediatric patients. Anesth Analg 89:1426-1429.
2. Rowe R, Andropoulos D, Heard M et al (1994) Anesthestic management of pediatric patients undergoing thoracoscopy. Cardiothorac Vasc Anesth 8:563.
3. Hammer G (2004) Single-lung ventilation in infants and children. Pediatric Anesthesia 14:98-102.
4. Golianu B, Hammer GB (2005) Pediatric thoracic anestesia. Curr Opin Anaesthesiol 18:5-11.
5. Disma N, Mameli L, Pini-Prato A, Montobbio G (2011) One lung ventilation with Arndt pediatric bronchial blocker for thoracoscopic surgery in children: a unicentric experience. Paediatr Anaesth 21:465-467.
6. Wald SH, Mahajan A, Kaplan MB, Atkinson JB (2005) Experience with the Arndt paediatric bronchial blocker. Br J Anaesth 94:92-94.
7. Campos J (2007) Which device should be considered the best for lung isolation: double-lumen endotracheal tube versus bronchial blockers. Curr Opin Anaesthesiol 20:27-31.
8. Campos J, Ezra A, Hallam BA et al (2006) Devices for Lung Isolation Used by Anesthesiologists with Limited Thoracic Experience. Comparison of Double-lumen Endotracheal Tube, Univent Torque Control Blocker, and Arndt Wire-guided Endobronchial Blocker. Anesthesiology 104:261-266.
9. Schmidt C, Rellensmann G, Van Aken H et al (2005) Single-Lung Ventilation for Pulmonary Lobe Resection in a Newborn. Anesth Analg 101:362-364.

Anesthesia Management in Severe Prematurity

15

Marinella Astuto and Concetta Gullo

15.1 Introduction

Over the last 30 years, greater numbers of premature infants of decreasing gestational age and extremely low birth weight (ELBW) have survived thanks to advances in neonatal intensive care and obstetrics. The increased survival of premature neonates has produced a population of infants who are susceptible to many unique diseases and a host of potential anesthetic challenges. With this increased survival rate, the need for infants to undergo surgery is not infrequent. It may be performed for surgical ligation of a patent ductus arteriosus (PDA), which is causing severe heart failure not controlled by medical therapy, or a laparotomy for the consequences of necrotizing enterocolitis (NEC).

These infants are also at risk of developing retinopathy of prematurity (ROP), which often coexists with chronic lung disease and may require laser or cryosurgery. Many develop inguinal hernias, which occur with increased frequency in those born before a gestational age of 32 weeks and a birth weight of less than1,250 g [1]. Inguinal hernia repair remains the most common surgical procedure carried out in pre-term infants. For the purpose of this chapter, we will focus on the very low and ELBW infant, or severe prematurity, and discuss the associated developmental physiology and its impact on anesthetic care.

15.2 Defining the Levels of Prematurity

Prematurity is defined as birth before 37 weeks of gestation, which is based on the last menstrual period and ultrasound scan. Unfortunately, ultrasonographic assess-

M. Astuto (✉)
Anesthesia and Intensive Care, Pediatric Anesthesia and Intensive Care Section,
and Postgraduate School, University of Catania, AOU Policlinico-Vittorio Emanuele
Catania, Italy

M. Astuto (ed.) *Pediatric Anesthesia, Intensive Care and Pain: Standardization
in Clinical Practice.* Anesthesia, Intensive Care and Pain in Neonates and Children
DOI: 10.1007/978-88-470-2685-8_15, © Springer-Verlag Italia 2013

ment of gestational age in the second trimester is not always accurate. An error of 1.2 weeks can have a significant impact on management decisions, because survival rate improves significantly with each incremental week of intrauterine life beyond 23 weeks of gestation [2]. Premature babies may be further divided into borderline prematurity (36–37 weeks of gestation), moderate prematurity (31–36 weeks of gestation), and severe prematurity (24–30 weeks of gestation) [3]. Low birth weight (LBW) infants are defined as infants born with a birth weight of less than 2,500 g; very low birth weight (VLBW) infants are those with a birth weight of less than 1,500 g; and ELBW infants are infants with a birth weight of less than 1,000 g. Birth weight may therefore be a more accurate measure of prematurity. In fact, comparisons between gestational age and birth weight have found them to be independent predictors of survival [4].

15.3 Problems Associated with Severely Premature and Extremely Low Birth Weight Infants

Morbidity and mortality for the smallest infants remains high with one study estimating a mortality rate of 89% for infants weighing 401–500 g. Almost all of the survivors in this ELBW group suffered from considerable morbidity [5].

The premature infant presents a unique physiology, anatomy, and pathology and requires focused strategies for presurgical management and for the administration of anesthesia. Most of the important organs in these babies are still in the process of development and maturation. There is inadequate production of efficient surfactant, a susceptibility of retinal blood vessels to oxygen toxicity, and a susceptibility to hemorrhagic and ischemic brain damage. These factors lead to the development of diseases exclusively found in these babies, e.g., respiratory distress syndrome (RDS), intraventricular hemorrhage, ROP, PDA, and NEC. Other factors include hypoglycemia, apnea (especially during the postoperative period), and hypothermia.

15.3.1 Pulmonary Disease

Premature infants of less than 32 weeks gestation are at increased risk of developing RDS. This is characterized by increasing atelectasis secondary to the inadequate production of surfactant. This low level of surfactant leads to alveolar collapse, a reduction in functional residual capacity, intrapulmonary shunting, and hyaline membrane formation. Atelectasis, hyaline membrane formation, and interstitial edema combine to reduce pulmonary compliance and necessitate the use of supplemental oxygen and positive pressure ventilation. The incidence and severity of RDS is inversely proportional to gestational age. Bronchopulmonary dysplasia (BPD) is defined as the need for supplemental oxygen before 30 days of life. BPD is a combination of pulmonary parenchymal and interstitial changes secondary to the effects of oxygen therapy and positive pressure ventilation on the premature lung. A severity index for BPD based on the need for supplemental oxygen and/or positive pressure ventilation or nasal continuous positive airway pressure has been developed, and shown to identify a spectrum of risk for adverse pulmonary and neurodevelopmental outcomes in prematurely born infants [6]. Anesthetic goals include minimizing the inspired oxygen concentration and peak inspiratory pressures while maintaining oxygenation and ventilation. The introduction of maternal steroid administration and artificial surfactant replacement therapy in the infant with less than 28 weeks gestational age has dramatically improved the prognosis of these infants.

15.3.2 Apnea and Respiratory Control

Severely premature infants possess a biphasic ventilatory response to hypoxia. Initially, ventilation increases during hypoxia, but after several minutes, ventilation decreases and apnea may ensue [7]. Apneic episodes occur commonly in the severely premature but decrease with advancing postconceptional age [8].

Apneic spells are a common neonatal problem occurring in approximately 25% of premature infants and ex pre-term infants during recovery from general anesthesia [9]. The apnea of prematurity and apnea following general anesthesia appear to have a similar distribution of central (70%), obstructive (10%), and mixed (20%) origins [10].

Pre-term infants with a history of periodic breathing often become apneic in response to airway obstruction; this effect declines with increasing postnatal age. As upper airway obstruction appears to be important in the development of apnea, it seems reasonable to assume that general anesthesia, which can decrease upper airway muscle tone, may contribute to the development of apnea after general anesthesia, even in infants without a history of apnea. Prolonged apnea is often accompanied by hypoxia, hypercarbia, and bradycardia. Apnea is usually defined as absent respiratory airflow of 15 s or longer. Postoperative apnea occurs as a cluster of episodes over several minutes, with minutes of normal breathing in between the clusters, accompanied by bradycardia. The incidence of postoperative apnea depends on postconceptional and gestational age, hematocrit, and the type of surgical procedure. The most significant risk factor is postconceptional age; the lower the postconceptional age, the greater the risk. Hypothermia and hypoglycemia are known to induce apnea. Anemia (hematocrit < 30%) and younger gestational age increase the risk of apnea for a given postconceptional age [11,12].

15.3.3 Brain Injury

Brain injury in premature infants includes intraventricular hemorrhage (IVH), cerebral ischemia [periventricular leukomalacia (PVL)], and posthemorrhagic hydrocephalus. IVH is the most common cause of intracranial hemorrhage in VLBW infants.

The incidence and severity of IVH is directly proportional to the degree of prematurity. An early onset of IVH appears during the first day of life. Risk factors include fetal distress, vaginal delivery, low Apgar (appearance, pulse, grimace, activity, respiration) scores, metabolic acidosis, hypercapnia, and the need for mechanical ventilation [13,14].

Hypercapnia, hypoglycemia, and anemia are associated with a rise in cerebral blood flow which may induce the onset of IVH. Factors that may decrease the incidence and severity of IVH include the administration of sedation with opioids, antenatal glucocorticoids, or indometacin. The outcome for infants with IVH depends, to a large extent, on the degree of associated parenchymal injury.

PVL is due to the impairment of the blood supply to the cerebral white matter. Severe hypotension, marked hypocarbia, and impairment of cerebral autoregulation in these infants are some of the risk factors leading to insufficient cerebral blood flow and ischemia.

15.3.4 Retinopathy of Prematurity

The pathophysiology of ROP is thought to be due to retinal artery constriction leading to retinal ischemia resulting in neovascularization. ROP occurs in approximately 50% of ELBW infants, with the incidence and severity being inversely proportional to birth weight and gestational age [15–17]. Although the pathogenesis of ROP is not completely understood, variations in arterial oxygenation (hypoxia or hyperoxia) and exposure to bright light appear to play a role.

One theory suggests that the combination of the hyperoxic vasoconstriction of retinal vessels, the induction of vascular endothelial growth factors, and free oxygen radicals damage the spindle cells in the retina. Other contributing factors include the use of supplemental oxygen, fluctuations in oxygen saturation, mechanical ventilation, total parenteral nutrition (TPN), and blood transfusion [18].

During anesthesia, the lowest inspired oxygen concentration that provides oxygen saturations between 92% and 96% is used and all attempts are made to avoid significant fluctuations in oxygen saturation.

15.3.5 Gastrointestinal Disease

NEC is an intestinal disease more common in premature infants and occurs in about 5% of ELBW infants; birth weight less than 1000 g that is the most important risk factor for NEC [19]. The prognosis for ELBW infants with NEC is poor. The pathogenesis of NEC has a multifactorial etiology, including hypoperfusion of the gut due to systemic hypoxia or hypotension, infection due to bacterial translocation across an immature gut wall, and enteric feeding, typically coincide with the onset of enteral feeding. Other factors include exposure to antenatal glucocorticoids, vaginal delivery, the need for mechanical ventilator support, PDA, exposure to postnatal indometacin, and a low Apgar score at 5 min [20].

The initial signs of NEC are feeding intolerance, increased work breathing, temperature instability, and lethargy; later signs include abdominal distension, bile-stained vomiting, bloody and frothy stools, gastric residuals of previous feeds, and periumbilical discoloration. There may be signs of systemic sepsis—circulatory collapse, hypotension, apnea, low blood glucose levels—and occasionally signs of gut perforation. Thrombocytopenia is common and may require correction. Initial management includes resuscitation, cardiopulmonary support, and antibiotics. Large volumes of colloids may be required together with blood and blood components. Surgical intervention may be required when there is perforation and when there is continuing deterioration despite full support.

15.3.6 Temperature Regulation

Premature and ELBW infants are susceptible to hypothermia during surgery. At birth, body temperature tends to decrease and this is due to heat loss from physical contact with cold surfaces or cold clothing as the temperature control system of premature infants is not yet developed. Moreover, the neonate depends on nonshivering thermogenesis for heat production. Nonshivering thermogenesis uses brown adipose tissue and requires oxygen consumption. It is believed that in small premature infants, brown adipose tissue is not sufficiently developed, and this, combined with the larger surface/volume ratio, makes infants more susceptible to hypothermia. In fact, brown fat cells begin to differentiate from reticular cells at 20 to 30 weeks of gestation and increase in size and number about 3–6 weeks after birth [3]. Volatile anesthetics are potent inhibitors of brown adipose tissue thermogenesis [21,22], while nitrous oxide and intravenous anesthetics such as sodium thiopental and propofol do not have this inhibitory property [23]. Hypothermia significantly increases metabolic activity and oxygen consumption, and this leads to serious clinical consequences such as hypoxemia, metabolic acidosis, periodic breathing or apnea, respiratory distress, bradycardia, hyperglycemia, and pulmonary aspiration of gastric contents, all factors that may seriously threaten the infant's life [3].

A premature infant's flaccid, open posture tends to increase heat loss rather than conserve heat, whereas the flexed, curled-up position of full-term neonates tends to conserve heat. We have to then add to this the risk in patients with central nervous system damage or suffering from hypoglycemia, who have more difficulty maintaining body temperature. After exposure to low temperatures, infants appear agitated because they increase their muscle activity in an attempt at compensation. This also produces an increase in the secretion of catecholamines in the serum as an attempt to increase heat production and safeguard the noble organs from the effects of hypothermia.

Both before arrival in the operating room and during any operation, heat loss must be minimized; therefore, any transport of the infant has to be in a thermo-heated incubator and an adequate temperature has to be maintained through the use of heat exchangers connected to special thermal blankets. It is of great importance to carefully cover the body of the infant, and in particular the head, which in this subject is a large surface for heat loss [3,24].

15.3.7 Patent Ductus Arteriosus

The PDA connects the main pulmonary artery with the aorta. It is essential during intrauterine life and its persistent patency is common in prematurity [25].

The small dimensions of the ducts result in a minimum left–right shunt without major hemodynamic consequences, while in the larger volume ducts overload will affect pulmonary circulation and the left sections over time, with the appearance of cyanosis and pulmonary hypertension.

In many cases, the duct closes spontaneously; where this does not happen, pharmacological intervention or surgery is necessary. The initial medical treatment includes fluid restriction [26–28], diuretics, and the administration of cyclooxygenase inhibitors, indometacin, and ibuprofen [28–30]. Indometacin therapy is less likely to close the PDA in ELBW infants compared with pre-term infants and is more likely to produce complications, including thrombocytopenia, renal failure, hyponatremia, and intestinal perforation [31].

Surgery consists of ligation through a left thoracotomy [32], with retraction of the left lung with decreased lung compliance. One of the most feared complications is severe bleeding [33]. When surgery is performed by experienced teams, the incidence of major complications is small [34].However, substantial late morbidity and mortality have been reported from the long-term complications of prematurity.

Anesthesia includes the use of fentanyl (20–50   g/kg) and pancuronium bromide (0.2 mg/kg). Although this procedure does not usually cause hypotension or bradycardia, a reduction in arterial pressure after anesthetic induction does occur because of loss of sympathetic tone, especially in the setting of hypovolemia due to diuretic therapy. This condition can be prevented by administering albumin (10 mL/kg) before induction [33].

15.3.8 Infection

Pneumonia, sepsis, and meningitis are the most common infections in *premature and ELBW infants*. The presence of catheters and respirators can, in fact, become a vehicle for bacteria. The main reason is that infants do not have a fully developed immune system, which is adapted to respond appropriately to external pathogens. The signs of sepsis are nonspecific and immediate; however, the following should be considered as possible signs of an infection: the presence of hypo- or hyperthermia, lethargy, apnea, or an increase of serum glucose levels. Sepsis can develop without changes in white blood cell count (WBC), fever, or signs of positive blood cell cultures. However, a 15% increase in WBC may be suggestive of an infection [35]. On occasions, traces of WBC in the cerebral spinal fluid and urine can be found [36].

Treatment with antibiotics appears to be the most appropriate therapy, even if aminoglycosides can cause muscle weakness and paralysis. Recent studies have shown that early treatment of sepsis is very important to prevent neurological damage from developing even several years after the original infection [37].

15.3.9 Anemia

Anemia is defined as a reduction of the total quantity of circulating hemoglobin in the peripheral blood and within erythrocytes. Premature infants are particularly subject to anemia because red blood cells in the neonatal period have a shorter life span and during the first weeks of life, their production is limited, being body growth relatively faster. At birth, the concentration of hematocrits (50–55%) is greater in infants than in older children and adults. This concentration tends to decrease normally in about in 2 or 3 months [3].

Normally, fetal hemoglobin is replaced by the adult variety which has lower affinity with oxygen (the affinity of hemoglobin for oxygen is a reduced P50 of 19 mmHg in the newborn vs. 30 mmHg in the infant vs. 27 mmHg in the adult). Consequently, in pre-term infants with the same hematocrit, less oxygen is delivered to the tissues. The situation can be aggravated by poor nutrition of the newborn with low vitamin E, folic acid, and iron, and by lung disorders [3,38].

In these premature infants, elective surgery should not take place when the hemoglobin concentration is lower than 10 g/dL. Thrombocytopenia occurs in about 70% of premature infants and the cause is not always very clear, although sepsis, coagulation intravascular disease, and NEC are among the most common causes. In the preoperative evaluation, a recent platelet count must be obtained and platelet availability must be evaluated [33]. The hematology values at different ages are shown in Table 15.1.

15.3.10 Hyperbilirubinemia

Almost all pre-term infants less than 35 weeks old have elevated levels of total bilirubin in serum or plasma and this condition is called prenatal jaundice. The

Table 15.1 Hematology values at different ages [68–70]

	Pre-term 28–32 weeks	Pre-term 32–36 weeks	Full-term infant
Hemoglobin (g/dL)	12.9	13.6	16.8
Hematocrit (%)	40.9	43.6	55
White blood cell count(/mm³)	5,160	7,710	18,000
Platelet count (/mm³)	255,000	260,000	300,000
Prothrombin time (s)	15.4	13	13
Activated partial thromboplastin time (s)	108	53.6	42.9
Fibrinogen (mg/dL)	256	243	283
Bleeding time (min)		3.5	3.5

yellowish discoloration of the skin and/or sclerae is caused by bilirubin deposition because pre-term infants have a reduced ability to conjugate this substance. The major complication produced by bilirubin is a neurological dysfunction (bilirubin-induced neurological dysfunction), which occurs when the circulating bilirubin crosses the blood–brain barrier and binds to brain tissue. A bilirubin concentration of 10–15 mg/dL causes kernicterus if the infant is in a state of acidosis and hypoxemia [39–41]. Additionally, certain substances such as sulfonamides, furosemide, and benzyl alcohol, having high affinity for proteins, displace bilirubin thereby increasing the risk of kernicterus [33]. Therefore, a two-volume exchange transfusion should be performed before surgery if the infant has elevated indirect bilirubin, because intraoperative hypoxemia and acidosis may prove disastrous.

15.3.11 Electrolyte Disorders

In the infant in a critical condition, the relationship between energy expenditure and water loss is affected by functional immaturity, environmental stress, and redistribution of body water at birth. The premature infant has a relative excess of the total volume of water and extracellular fluid than the full-term infant. Changes in the concentration of electrolytes in the premature infant can be very frequent, but one should never rely on the first sample [42]. An increase of sodium in the blood may be caused either by excessive dehydration or by the excessive administration of sodium [3]. Renal blood flow and glomerular filtration rate (GFR) increase with gestational age; in full-term newborns, these parameters improve rapidly after birth, while they remain altered in premature infants, resulting in intolerance to excessive fluid and electrolytes [42]. Hypokalemia is common (< 3 mEq/L), especially in pre-term infants who received diuretics. The serum chloride concentration is normally higher (105–115 mEq/L) and the total calcium concentration is usually lower than that of full-term infants. Hyperventilation may further reduce serum potassium levels and ionized calcium concentration.

Most neonatologists tend to maintain the total serum calcium concentration above 8 mg/dL, although many neonates do perfectly well with concentrations below this level [3]. The serum calcium concentration in premature and ELBW infants is normally lower than that of full-term infants because pre-term infants have a diminished concentration of serum proteins [3].

15.3.12 Hypoglycemia

Premature and LBW infants are susceptible to hypoglycemia. This is attributed to immature gluconeogenic and glycogenolytic enzyme systems. A plasma glucose concentration of less than 25 mg/dL in these infants is taken as a sign of hypoglycemia. Infants who use glucose at an increased rate are prone to hypoglycemia, e.g., infants experiencing perinatal asphyxia, neonatal sepsis, and a cold environment [43].

Glucose levels in infants at increased risk of hypoglycemia should be checked intraoperatively. Intravenous infusions should contain glucose to maintain a glucose infusion rate of between 6 and 8 mg/kg/min.

15.4 Anesthetic Management

Anesthesia provides insensitivity to pain during surgical procedures. The most commonly used technique in severely premature infants is general anesthesia. Over the last 25 years, general anesthesia has been delivered using both inhaled and intravenous drugs in very premature infants for a variety of surgical procedures. The most frequent diseases for which surgery is required in VLBW infants are inguinal hernia, NEC, PDA, ROP, and ventriculoperitoneal shunt.

15.5 Drug Pharmacokinetics and Pharmacodynamics

The pharmacokinetics and pharmacodynamics of drugs for severe premature infants are different from those of full-term neonates, children, or adults.

The main factors affecting drug pharmacokinetics in severely premature infants are higher body water than body fat content, which results in higher volume distribution, and hence a need for a higher loading dose, and a decrease in albumin and α1-acid glycoprotein binding leading to an increase in free drug concentration. In these infants, the biotransformation of drugs by hepatic enzyme systems may be slower due to the immaturity of the systems. Renal excretion of drugs may be slow or impaired due to low renal blood flow, low GFR, and poor tubular secretion. The minimum alveolar concentration of inhaled anesthetics is lower in pre-term infants compared with full-term neonates [44].

15.6 Effects of Anesthesia and Sedation on Brain Development

Recent findings in neonatal animals have revealed that all commonly used anesthetics and sedatives induce neuronal cell death in several regions of the developing brain [45,46].

Whether the observed degenerating neurons were destined to die by physiologically programmed cell death, called apoptosis, or whether exposure to the anesthetic induced apoptotic cell death in neurons otherwise not destined to die remains controversial [47]. Nonetheless, these disturbing findings in animals have raised significant safety concerns regarding anesthetic exposure in immature neonates [48].

Emerging findings from epidemiological studies in humans remain conflicting; while some studies have suggested an association between anesthetic exposure early in life and subsequent learning or behavioral abnormalities [49,50], other studies have failed to find this association [51,52]. The mechanism for neurotoxicity appears to be attributed to the neurotransmitters glutamate and γ-aminobutyric acid, which act as trophic factors in the developing brain [53]. In the immature brain, these trophic factors promote synaptic growth and plasticity and are necessary for neuronal survival.

The inhaled anesthetics ketamine, nitrous oxide, and midazolam exert their anesthetic effects by altering synaptic transmission through the blockade of glutamate and γ-aminobutyric acid receptors. In the immature brain, this blockade also precipitates neuronal cell death by apoptosis [54]. Moreover, pre-term infants who receive anesthesia and sedation for painful procedures experience less morbidity and mortality than those who do not [55,56]. Based on animal models, the severe premature infant exposed to several hours of high concentrations of the inhaled anesthetics ketamine, nitrous oxide, and midazolam is potentially at risk, as is the premature infant exposed to surgery with insufficient anesthesia. We often anesthetize babies with low concentrations of the inhaled agent, but with large doses of opioids and regional anesthesia whenever possible.

15.7   Choice of Operation Site

Which is the best place to perform surgery in severe premature infants, the operating room or the neonatal intensive care unit (NICU)?

Anesthesiologists and surgeons are more comfortable performing surgery in an operating room which allows them to work in a familiar place with access to the assistance of colleagues and nursing staff, and a variety of surgical and anesthetic equipment nearby. On the other hand, performing surgery in the NICU avoids transportation of the infant which may be accompanied by a significant amount of risk.

In the past, some surgeons chose to perform surgery at the bedside in the NICU without an anesthesiologist present because it was deemed unsafe to transport the infant, or if there was no operating room or anesthesiologist to perform the surgery in a timely manner, or because it was believed that the severely premature did not need anesthesia. In the authors' opinion, this model of care does not provide the highest level of patient care; there is ample evidence that premature neonates require anesthesia for surgery.

There is clearly no answer as to which is the best place. The decision should be made based on the setting and conditions in each individual case and institution, minimizing the period of transportation and providing optimal surgical conditions (optimal lighting, sterile conditions, and controlled room temperature).

15.8 Preoperative Evaluation

Preoperative preparation focuses on the optimization of cardiac and respiratory status and on the treatment of anemia, electrolyte abnormalities, metabolic acidosis, and coagulopathy. For nonemergency procedures such as inguinal hernia repair, preoperative evaluation occurs well in advance of surgery to optimize medical status before the administration of anesthesia. Communication between the anesthesiologist, surgeon, and neonatologist before and after surgery is vital for safe care. For almost all surgeries, packed red blood cells should be available in the operating room.

The NPO (nil by mouth) status should be determined. In our institution, babies less than 6 months are required to be NPO for formula for 4 h or longer, breast milk for 3 h or longer, and clear liquids for 2 h or longer (Table 15.2)

15.9 General Anesthesia

Anesthesia may be induced using either an inhalational agent or an intravenous agent; usually this depends on whether the infant has an intravenous catheter in place and whether there is a risk of pulmonary aspiration. For elective procedures, inhalation induction of anesthesia is common because access may be difficult after a long neonatal NICU stay. Saphenous, external jugular, and scalp veins often yield the greatest success when it is impossible to insert a hand or foot intravenous cannula. The size of the endotracheal tube (ETT) chosen should be based on the age of the infant and whether they require prolonged tracheal intubation (> 1 months) in the NICU. If the infant has to undergo a prolonged period of tracheal intubation, the ETT used should have an internal diameter that is 0.5 mm smaller than the tube usually chosen for a child of this age. The anesthesiologist should ensure that there is an adequate air leak around the ETT during positive pressure ventilation to prevent an excessively tight tube from contributing to postoperative tracheal edema and airway obstruction.

Particular intraoperative concerns for severely premature infants include maintenance of normal body temperature, balanced use of intravenous fluids, and effective humidification of inhaled gases to promote effective pulmonary hygiene and help maintain a normal body temperature. Premature infants have large surface area/volume ratios and lose body heat easily through their skin. For infants less than 6 months of age, the operating room should be pre-warmed to prevent radiant heat loss during preparation and before the young patient is covered with drapes. A warming mattress, a heated and humidified breathing circuit, and warmed intravenous fluids further help prevent heat loss. A reduction of body temperature contributes

Table 15.2 Preoperative fasting recommendations in infants and children

Age	Formula	Breast milk	Clear liquids
< 6 months	4 h	3 h	2 h

to an increase in the expenditure of metabolic energy postoperatively and may contribute to apnea in infants of less than 60 weeks postconceptional age.

Intravenous fluids consist primarily of a balanced salt solution (such as lactated Ringer's solution) for the replacement of intraoperative fluid losses. The compositions of commonly used intravenous solutions are shown in Table 15.3.

Maintenance fluids need not contain dextrose routinely, but should be used for patients receiving continuous infusion via TPN or those with documented hypoglycemia. For the smallest premature infants (< 3 months of age) who have inadequate glycogen stores, the routine administration of a 5–10% dextrose solution at maintenance rates will usually maintain normal blood glucose concentrations. Maintenance fluid rate can be calculate as 4 mL/kg/h for the first 10 kg of body weight plus 2 mL/kg/h for the next 10 kg of body weight plus 1 mL/kg/h for each kg thereafter (Table 15.4).

Positioning of the patient must be done in a way that prevents hyperextension of contracted joints. Placing a roll under the infant's upper back will align the airway of infants with large heads relative to their chest size.

The hemodynamic state should be maintained in as stable a level as possible to avoid an abrupt increase or decrease in cerebral blood flow, which may lead to intracerebral hemorrhage or cerebral ischemia. An estimate of the circulating blood volume is shown in Table 15.5.

Table 15.3 Composition of extracellular fluid and commonly used intravenous solutions

	Na^+	K^+	Ca^{2+}	Mg^{2+}	NH_4^+	Cl^-	HCO_3^-	HPO_4^-
Extracellular fluid	142	4	5	3	0.3	103	27	3
Lactated Ringer's solution	130	4	3	–	–	109	28	–
0.45% NaCl	77	–	–	–	–	77	–	–
0.9% NaCl (normal saline)	154	–	–	–	–	154	–	–
3% NaCl	590	–	–	–	–	590	–	–

Table 15.4 Maintenance fluid requirements in children

Weight (kg)	Hour	Day
< 10	4 mL/kg	100 mL/kg
10–20	40 mL + 2 mL/kg for every kg > 10 kg	1,000 mL + 50 mL/kg for every kg > 10 kg
> 20	60 mL + 1 mL/kg for every kg > 20 kg	1,500 mL + 20 mL/kg for every kg > 20 kg

Table 15.5 Estimate of circulating blood volume

Age	Estimated blood volume (mL/kg)
Pre-term infant	100
Full-term neonate	90
Infant	80
School age	75

Basic monitoring includes electrocardiogram, blood pressure, pulse oximetry, end-tidal carbon dioxide and temperature. For major surgery, invasive blood pressure monitoring, central venous pressure, and urine output may be needed. An intra-arterial cannula may be sited at the umbilical artery, radial artery, or posterior tibial artery.

15.10 Regional Anesthesia

There is increasing evidence that regional anesthesia is beneficial when used alone or in combination with general anesthesia in VLBW infants. Epidural anesthesia has been shown to decrease the need for postoperative ventilatory support in infants undergoing major surgery [57]. Huang and Hirshberg [58] showed that regional anesthesia decreased the need for postoperative mechanical ventilation in infants with a mean gestational age of 26 weeks and a mean postconceptional age at surgery of 38 weeks, when undergoing hernia repair. Good success rates and low complication rates have also been reported [59]. The incidence of postoperative apnea following general anesthesia has been reported to be 11–37%, whereas the risk of postoperative apnea following spinal anesthesia without sedative supplementation is close to 0% [60,61]. The risk of apnea, oxygen desaturation, and bradycardia is not completely abolished by the use of regional anesthesia because there is occasional need to supplement regional anesthesia with intravenous or inhaled agents.

Inguinal hernia repair is the most common surgical indication for regional anesthesia in severely premature infants. Inguinal hernia repair under spinal [62] or caudal [63,64] anesthesia is reported to have fewer episodes of apnea, hypoxemia, and bradycardia than in infants who receive general anesthesia [65]. The jury is out, though, because recent publications using newer inhalational agents (desflurane, sevoflurane) suggest little difference [66,67]. The main limitation of spinal anesthesia is the limited duration of action of local anesthetics, even when relatively large doses per kg of body weight are administered. The duration of action is up to 80% shorter in the youngest children compared with adults. The maximum duration of spinal anesthesia is about 90 min, even when long-acting local anesthetics are administered in relatively large doses. The short duration of action of intrathecal drugs in these infants has prompted interest in continuous regional anesthesia techniques so that the duration of anesthesia may be extended while drug toxicity is minimized. Successful regional anesthesia techniques offer many advantage in this high-risk population.

15.11 Emergence from Anesthesia

Extremely premature and VLBW infants who were mechanically ventilated before surgery should remain ventilated during the return journey to the NICU. The trachea need not be extubated in the operating room immediately after the surgical procedure even if the infant was not on a ventilator before surgery. The trachea can be extubated later in the NICU when full recovery from the remaining effects of the anesthetic is obtained.

15.12 Postoperative Management

Pre-term infants tend to have apneic spells postoperatively. The generally accepted limit of such a risk in infants is a 44–46 weeks postconceptional age. Monitors should be applied to detect apnea, desaturation, and bradycardia in these infants for at least 48 h postoperatively.

15.13 Conclusions

Severely premature and VLBW infants present significant challenges to the anesthesiologist. They are susceptible to prematurity-related diseases. When providing anesthesia for these infants, precautions should be taken to deliver safe anesthesia. Attention should be paid to the inspired oxygen concentration to avoid hyperoxia, which is a major contributing factor to the development of ROP. Hemodynamic parameters should be kept stable to avoid IVH and cerebral ischemia. Prevention of hypothermia and hypoglycemia is also essential. These infants handle drugs in a less predictable fashion and therefore there is a need to titrate drug dosages. These very young patients will benefit from adequate anesthesia and analgesia.

References

1. Peevy KJ, FA Speed, CJ Hoff (1986) Epidemiology of inguinal hernia in preterm neonates. Pediatrics, 77(2):246-247
2. Boat AC et al (2011) Outcome for the extremely premature neonate: how far do we push the edge? Paediatr Anaesth, 21(7):765-770
3. Gregory, ed. Pediatric Anestesia
4. El-Metwally D, B Vohr, R Tucker, (2000) Survival and neonatal morbidity at the limits of viability in the mid 1990s: 22 to 25 weeks. J Pediatr, 137(5):616-622
5. Lemons JA et al (2001) Very low birth weight outcomes of the National Institute of Child health and human development neonatal research network, January 1995 through December 1996. NICHD Neonatal Research Network. Pediatrics 107(1):E1
6. Kurth CD et al (1987) Postoperative apnea in preterm infants. Anesthesiology 66(4):483-488
7. Rigatto H, JP Brady (1972)Periodic breathing and apnea in preterm infants. II. Hypoxia as a primary event. Pediatrics 50(2):219-228
8. Daily WJ, M Klaus, HB Meyer (1969) Apnea in premature infants: monitoring, incidence, heart rate changes, and an effect of environmental temperature. Pediatrics, 43(4):510-518

9. Gallagher, TM and PM Crean, (1989) Spinal anaesthesia in infants born prematurely. Anaesthesia 44(5):434-436
10. Kurth CD, SE LeBard (1991) Association of postoperative apnea, airway obstruction, and hypoxemia in former premature infants. Anesthesiology 75(1):22-26
11. Cote CJ et al (1995) Postoperative apnea in former preterm infants after inguinal herniorrhaphy. A combined analysis. Anesthesiology 82(4):809-822
12. Welborn LG et al (1991) Anemia and postoperative apnea in former preterm infants. Anesthesiology 74(6):1003-1006
13. Wells JT, LR Ment, (1995).Prevention of intraventricular hemorrhage in preterm infants. Early Hum Dev 42(3):209-233
14. Kaiser JR et al (2006) Hypercapnia during the first 3 days of life is associated with severe intraventricular hemorrhage in very low birth weight infants. J Perinatol 26(5):279-285
15. Lermann VL, JB Fortes Filho, RS Procianoy (2006) The prevalence of retinopathy of prematurity in very low birth weight newborn infants. J Pediatr (Rio J), 82(1):27-32
16. Whitfill CR, AV Drack (2000) Avoidance and treatment of retinopathy of prematurity. Semin Pediatr Surg 9(2):103-105
17. Nair PM et al (2003) Retinopathy of prematurity in VLBW and extreme LBW babies. Indian J Pediatr 70(4):303-306
18. Cunningham S et al (1995) Transcutaneous oxygen levels in retinopathy of prematurity. Lancet 346(8988):1464-1465
19. Snyder CL et al (1997) Survival after necrotizing enterocolitis in infants weighing less than 1,000 g: 25 years' experience at a single institution. J Pediatr Surg 32(3):434-437
20. Guthrie SO et al (2003) Necrotizing enterocolitis among neonates in the United States. J Perinatol 23(4):278-285
21. Ohlson K.B et al (1994) Thermogenesis in brown adipocytes is inhibited by volatile anesthetic agents. A factor contributing to hypothermia in infants? Anesthesiology 81(1):176-183
22. Dicker A et al (1995) Halothane selectively inhibits nonshivering thermogenesis. Possible implications for thermoregulation during anesthesia of infants. Anesthesiology 82(2):491-501
23. Ohlson KB et al (2003) Thermogenesis inhibition in brown adipocytes is a specific property of volatile anesthetics. Anesthesiology 98(2):437-448
24. Jahnukainen T et al (1993) Dynamics of vasomotor thermoregulation of the skin in term and preterm neonates. Early Hum Dev 33(2):133-143
25. Trus T et al (1993) Optimal management of patent ductus arteriosus in the neonate weighing less than 800 g. J Pediatr Surg 28(9):1137-1379
26. Radtke WA, (1998)Current therapy of the patent ductus arteriosus. Curr Opin Cardiol 13(1):59-65
27. Stevenson JG (1977) Fluid administration in the association of patent ductus arteriosus complicating respiratory distress syndrome. J Pediatr 90(2):257-261
28. Heymann MA, AM Rudolph, NH Silverman (1976) Closure of the ductus arteriosus in premature infants by inhibition of prostaglandin synthesis. N Engl J Med 295(10):530-533
29. Merritt TA et al (1978) Closure of the patent ductus arteriosus with ligation and indomethacin: a consecutive experience. J Pediatr 93(4):639-646
30. Ohlsson A, R Walia, S Shah (2008) Ibuprofen for the treatment of patent ductus arteriosus in preterm and/or low birth weight infants. Cochrane Database Syst Rev (1):CD003481
31. Little DC et al (2009) Patent ductus arteriosus in micropreemies and full-term infants: the relative merits of surgical ligation versus indomethacin treatment. J Pediatr Surg 2003. 38(3):492-496
32. Benjacholmas V et al (2009) Short-term outcome of PDA ligation in the preterm infants at King Chulalongkorn Memorial Hospital, Thailand. J Med Assoc Thai 92(7):909-913
33. Cotè-Lerman-Todres (2003) Practice of Anesthesia in Infants and Children IV edition
34. Gould DS et al (2003) A comparison of on-site and off-site patent ductus arteriosus ligation in premature infants. Pediatrics 112(6 Pt 1):1298-1301

35. Spector SA, W Ticknor, M Grossman (1981) Study of the usefulness of clinical and hematologic findings in the diagnosis of neonatal bacterial infections. Clin Pediatr (Phila) 20(6):385-392
36. Avery GB (1988) Neonatology in the NICU: three new techniques, three continuing problems. Pediatr Ann 17(8):503
37. Schlapbach LJ et al (2011) Impact of sepsis on neurodevelopmental outcome in a Swiss National Cohort of extremely premature infants. Pediatrics 128(2):e348-357
38. Jilani T, MP Iqb al (2011) Does vitamin E have a role in treatment and prevention of anemia? Pak J Pharm Sci 24(2):237-242
39. Watchko JF, FA Oski (1992) Kernicterus in preterm newborns: past, present, and future. Pediatrics 90(5):707-715
40. Gartner LM et al (1970) Kernicterus: high incidence in premature infants with low serum bilirubin concentrations. Pediatrics 45(6):906-917
41. Okumura A et al (2009) Kernicterus in preterm infants. Pediatrics 123(6):e1052-1058
42. Parigi GB, chirurgia pediatrica Masson
43. Lorenz JM (2001) The outcome of extreme prematurity. Semin Perinatol 25(5):348-359
44. LeDez K.M, J Lerman (1987) The minimum alveolar concentration (MAC) of isoflurane in preterm neonates. Anesthesiology 67(3):301-307
45. Loepke AW, FX McGowan Jr, SG Soriano (2008) CON: The toxic effects of anesthetics in the developing brain: the clinical perspective. Anesth Analg 106(6):1664-1669
46. Loepke AW (2010) Developmental neurotoxicity of sedatives and anesthetics: a concern for neonatal and pediatric critical care medicine? Pediatr Crit Care Med 11(2):217-226
47. Loepke AW et al (2009).The effects of neonatal isoflurane exposure in mice on brain cell viability, adult behavior, learning, and memory. Anesth Analg, 108(1):90-104
48. Jevtovic-Todorovic V, JW Olney (2008) PRO: Anesthesia-induced developmental neuroapoptosis: status of the evidence. Anesth Analg 106(6):1659-1663
49. DiMaggio C et al (2009) A retrospective cohort study of the association of anesthesia and hernia repair surgery with behavioral and developmental disorders in young children. J Neurosurg Anesthesiol 21(4):286-291
50. Wilder RT et al (2009) Early exposure to anesthesia and learning disabilities in a population-based birth cohort. Anesthesiology 110(4):796-804
51. Sprung J et al (2009) Anesthesia for cesarean delivery and learning disabilities in a population-based birth cohort. Anesthesiology 111(2):302-310
52. Bartels M, RR Althoff, DI Boomsma (2009) Anesthesia and cognitive performance in children: no evidence for a causal relationship. Twin Res Hum Genet 12(3):246-253
53. Ikonomidou C et al (2001) Neurotransmitters and apoptosis in the developing brain. Biochem Pharmacol 62(4):401-405
54. Ikonomidou C et al (1999) Blockade of NMDA receptors and apoptotic neurodegeneration in the developing brain. Science 283(5398):70-74
55. Anand KJ (2000) Pain, plasticity, and premature birth: a prescription for permanent suffering? Nat Med 6(9):971-973
56. Anand K.S (1993) Relationships between stress responses and clinical outcome in newborns, infants, and children. Crit Care Med 21(9 Suppl):S358-S359
57. Bosenberg AT (1998) Epidural analgesia for major neonatal surgery. Paediatr Anaesth 8(6):479-483
58. Huang JJ, G Hirshberg (2001) Regional anaesthesia decreases the need for postoperative mechanical ventilation in very low birth weight infants undergoing herniorrhaphy. Paediatr Anaesth 11(6):705-709
59. Webster AC et al (1993) Lumbar epidural anaesthesia for inguinal hernia repair in low birth weight infants. Can J Anaesth 40(7):670-675
60. Welborn LG et al (1990) Postoperative apnoea in former preterm infants: does anaemia increase the risk? Can J Anaesth 37(4 Pt 2):S92

61. Veverka TJ et al (1991) Spi nal anesthesia reduces the hazard of apnea in high-risk infants. Am Surg 57(8):531-534; discussion 534-535
62. Krane EJ, CM Haberkern, LE Jacobson (1995) Postoperative apnea, bradycardia, and oxygen desaturation in formerly premature infants: prospective comparison of spinal and general anesthesia. Anesth Analg 80(1):7-13
63. Hoelzle M et al (2010) Comparison of awake spinal with awake caudal anesthesia in preterm and ex-preterm infants for herniotomy. Paediatr Anaesth 20(7):620-624
64. Walther-Larsen S, LS Rasmussen (2006) The former preterm infant and risk of post-operative apnoea: recommendations for management. Acta Anaesthesiol Scand 50(7):888-893
65. Steward DJ (1982) Preterm infants are more prone to complications following minor surgery than are term infants. Anesthesiology, 56(4):304-306
66. Somri M et al (1998) Postoperative outcome in high-risk infants undergoing herniorrhaphy: comparison between spinal and general anaesthesia. Anaesthesia 53(8):762-766
67. Sale SM et al (2006) Prospective comparison of sevoflurane and desflurane in formerly premature infants undergoing inguinal herniotomy. Br J Anaesth 96(6):774-778
68. Andrew M (1997) The relevance of developmental hemostasis to hemorrhagic disorders of newborns. Semin Perinatol 21:70–85
69. Andrew M, Vegh P, Johnston M, et al (1992) Maturation of the hemostatic system during childhood. Blood 80:1998–2005
70. Goodnight SH, Hathaway WE (2001) Disorders of Hemostasis and Thrombosis, A Clinical Guide, 2nd ed. New York, McGraw-Hill, pp 31-38

Emergence Delirium: Assessment, Prevention, and Decision-Making

16

Pablo Mauricio Ingelmo, Carmelo Minardi,
Stefano Scalia Catenacci and Andrew J. Davidson

16.1   Definition

Agitation or delirium during early emergence from anesthesia was first described in the 1960s [1,2]. Smessaert and colleagues [1] described three types of recovery from anesthesia: (1) patients with a tranquil and uneventful recovery; (2) patients who showed a moderate degree of restlessness; and (3) patients who were markedly delirious and uncooperative, and who required special care and restraint. They also described two main causative factors for postanesthetic delirium. The first was related to the anesthetic (cyclopropane more so than ether or barbiturates) and surgical procedures (peripheral surgery less so than intrathoracic or intra-abdominal surgery), and the second was related to the individual characteristics of the patient (e.g., sex, age, and mental attitude). They finally hypothesized that emergence from surgical anesthesia was primarily influenced by the patient's personality and that pain was not the essential factor causing delirium [1].

Eckenhoff and colleagues [2] also reported signs of hyperexcitation in patients emerging from ether, cyclopropane, or ketamine anesthesia, particularly when administered for tonsillectomy, thyroidectomy, and circumcision. In these cases, children experienced postanesthesia agitation more often than adults [1].

Halothane was the predominant anesthetic for decades; when combined with adequate postoperative pain management, the incidence of emergence agitation (EA) was attenuated [3]. However, with the introduction of sevoflurane and desflurane, the incidence of EA appeared to increase. It was noted that children suddenly entered a state of excitation in which they could not be consoled by the usual methods [4].

Postoperative negative behaviors in children include a variety of clinical conditions ranging from crying and irritability to severe agitation, disorientation, or even

P.M. Ingelmo (✉)
First Service of Anesthesia and Intensive Care
San Gerardo Hospital, Monza, Italy
e-mail: pabloingelmo@libero.it

M. Astuto (ed.) *Pediatric Anesthesia, Intensive Care and Pain: Standardization in Clinical Practice.* Anesthesia, Intensive Care and Pain in Neonates and Children
DOI: 10.1007/978-88-470-2685-8_16, © Springer-Verlag Italia 2013

delirium. The terms "emergence excitement" and "EA" are often used in the literature as alternate terms to describe delirium symptomatology [5,6].

Emergence delirium (ED) has been inadequately defined in the literature and a number of terms have been used interchangeably, including EA and paradoxical excitement. ED has been defined as a mental disorder in which children are crying, thrashing about, are inconsolable, uncooperative, and show signs of delusions, confusion, hallucinations, and paranoid ideation during early emergence from anesthesia [7]. Sikich and Lerman defined ED as "a mental disturbance during the recovery from general anesthesia consisting of hallucinations, delusions and confusion manifested by moaning, restlessness, involuntary physical activity, and thrashing about in bed [8]." The standard diagnostic criteria for delirium are a disturbance in consciousness or awareness (demonstrated by a reduced awareness of the environment and an inability to focus attention) associated with changes in cognition (such as disorientation) or perceptual disturbances [9]. In the context of postoperative ED, the delirium is usually associated with a motor component such as restlessness or thrashing about. In contrast, EA is a state of restlessness and mental distress and can arise from a number of sources including pain, physiological compromise, or anxiety. Not all children that have EA have delirium. A child may be agitated for numerous reasons including pain, hunger, or fear, or because of the absence of a primary caregiver or unfamiliar surroundings. "Agitation" can be used as a general term that encompasses all of these states, but it should be avoided in publications that specifically discuss the ED phenomenon [9].

The majority of publications that investigate ED or EA do not clearly indicate if the phenomenon measured is ED or EA. This is partly because most of the scales used cannot clearly differentiate between the two. This has led to considerable contradictions over the true incidence, causative factors, and appropriate treatment for ED. For example, the quoted incidence of ED ranges from 10 to 80%, depending on the studies. The most frequently quoted incidence is probably about 20% [10,11].

ED usually occurs within the first 30 min after anesthesia and is self-limiting after 5–15 min [10,12–14].

It can be a serious problem and may cause self-injury of the child or accidental removal of intravenous catheters, and may require extra nursing care and supplemental sedative or analgesic drugs. ED also reduces parental and caregiver satisfaction [5,10]. The long-term psychological implications of ED are unclear, but it has been shown that children who show ED while emerging from anesthesia have a higher risk of developing separation anxiety, apathy, and sleep and eating disorders up to 2 weeks after surgery [15].

16.2 Associated Factors

The etiology of ED is currently unknown. As mentioned previously, research into the etiology and management of ED has been hampered by a lack of clear consensus regarding its definition [9]. Recent hypotheses emphasize that rapid emergence associated with sevoflurane and desflurane may create a dissociative state with altered cognitive perception [16]. Sevoflurane has intrinsic effects that may contribute to ED. It has been noted that the electroencephalograph pattern in children anesthetized with sevoflurane differs from the pattern in children anesthetized with halothane [17] and may account for the different emergence characteristics.

Several factors have been associated with an increased risk of ED, including the child's baseline temperament and anxiety levels, parental presence, sevoflurane or desflurane anesthesia, age, postoperative pain, and ear, nose, and throat (ENT) procedures [18].

16.2.1 Sevoflurane and Desflurane Anesthesia vs Halothane Anesthesia

Sevoflurane and desflurane, agents with a low blood/gas solubility, have been associated with a higher incidence of ED and agitation when compared with halothane [19]. A meta-analysis of randomized controlled trials (RCTs) that compared the incidence of EA in children after sevoflurane and halothane anesthesia indicated that sevoflurane results in a higher probability (odds ratio 2.21, 95% confidence interval: 1.8–2.8) of EA than halothane. Desflurane has also been found to cause a high incidence of ED and agitation compared with halothane [16,20]. It has been suggested that recovery of consciousness after sevoflurane and desflurane may be very rapid, resulting in an accelerated and turbulent emergence in which postoperative analgesia may not be effective due to a misperception of environmental stimuli [17].

16.2.2 Sevoflurane vs. Desflurane

The incidence of ED reported in studies comparing sevoflurane and desflurane anesthesia varied between 10 and 55%. Welborn and colleagues [20] studied children undergoing ENT surgery and reported an incidence of ED of 55% after desflurane anesthesia compared with a 10% incidence of ED in children receiving sevoflurane. Pain may have been a contributing factor in this study, as opiates were not administered during surgery and the child's behavior after awakening was classified only as either "agitated" or "non-agitated". Cohen and colleagues [21] studied 100 preschool children undergoing adenotonsillectomy and receiving fentanyl 2.5 µg/kg during induction. They evaluated postoperative behavior using a three-point scale (calm, agitated but consolable, very agitated and inconsolable). The incidence of postoperative agitation was broadly similar after sevoflurane (18%) or desflurane (24%) anesthesia. Demirbilek and colleagues [22] reported similar results within a similar clinical setting and using the same methodology. Valley and colleagues [23] used the scale described by Cohen [21] to evaluate the postoperative behavior of children under 13 years of age who received sevoflurane or desflurane anesthesia combined with a caudal block. They found a 33% overall incidence of ED without significant differences between children receiving sevoflurane or desflurane anesthesia. None of these studies used a validated tool to assess postoperative behavior and may have described EA or pain instead of ED.

16.2.3 Sevoflurane and Desflurane Anesthesia vs. Propofol Anesthesia

Children receiving sevoflurane and desflurane anesthesia have an increased incidence and intensity of ED compared with those receiving propofol anesthesia [24]. In one particular study looking at children undergoing eye examinations, those receiving sevoflurane had an incidence of ED of 38% compared to 0% for those who had received propofol [5].

An initial explanation suggested that because awakening times correlate inversely with Pediatric Anesthesia Emergence Delirium (PAED) scores, a rapid awakening after sevoflurane anesthesia could cause this difference on ED [8,25]. However, the incidence of ED was higher after sevoflurane anesthesia even in the presence of similar awakening times [5,26]. Moreover, Oh and colleagues demonstrated that, even when obtaining a slow emergence by a gradual de-escalation of sevoflurane, the incidences of ED were did not decrease [27].

In contrast, Pieters and colleagues [28] and Konig and colleagues [29] suggested that, when measured with a validated score, there were no differences on the intensity of ED between sevoflurane or propofol anesthesia. However, both sudies reported that children receiving sevoflurane anesthesia received significantly more analgesic drugs in the postanesthesia care unit (PACU).

16.2.4 Type of Surgery

Otorhinolaryngologic surgery is an independent risk factor for ED [25]. Children undergoing head and neck surgery could experience a sense of suffocation on emergence and this could be the cause of increased agitation after awakening. Ophthalmologic surgery was also associated with an increased incidence of agitation or delirium during early emergence from anesthesia [30]. Blurred vision and/or ocular bandages may result in a perception of a hostile environment during awakening.

16.2.5 The Children and Their Parents

Children who develop ED are usually younger, manifest preoperative anxiety, are more emotional and impulsive, have reduced ability to adapt, and have parents who are more anxious [13,31]. The incidence of ED after sevoflurane anesthesia was greater for children whose ages were between 3 and 5 years compared with children whose ages were between 6 and 10 years [32].

Baseline temperament and anxiety levels in children have been seen to be associated with the occurrence of EA. Increased anxiety in the preoperative holding area as well as on induction of anesthesia have been associated with the development of maladaptive behavior during the postoperative period [31]. Voepel-Lewis and colleagues [14] found that temperament, as evidenced by low adaptability, was associated with EA.

A difficult separation from the parents before surgery is associated with a higher risk of ED [33]. Although RCTs evaluating the effects on the quality of emergence are scarce, some case-control studies suggest that the presence of parents during awakening may promote a better emergence environment, thus reducing any incidence of ED [34]. Demirbilek and colleagues suggested that fentanyl 2.5 µg/kg did not produce further reduction in the incidence of ED when associated with preoperative anxiety, adequate analgesia, and parental presence on awakening [22].

16.2.6 Postoperative Pain

Postoperative pain may be a significant contributing factor for EA or ED when assessing the cause of a child's behavior on emergence. However, it must be noted that a clear relationship has not been established. Inadequate pain relief may be the cause of agitation, particularly after short surgical procedures for which the peak effects of analgesics may be delayed until the child is completely awake [3,25,35].

It has been postulated that better pain control should result in a lower incidence of postoperative delirium. The administration of different types of analgesic drugs has been shown to reduce the agitation associated with sevoflurane anesthesia in children undergoing otorhinolaryngologic surgery, suggesting a potential relationship between pain and EA [14].

However, several studies in presumably pain-free patients have demonstrated a consistent incidence of EA, which suggests that analgesics cannot completely attenuate postanesthetic agitation [14,36]. Moreover, children who receive sevoflurane while undergoing diagnostic procedures without nociceptive stimulation (magnetic resonance imaging), presented with a significant incidence of ED [11].

16.3   Identification and Quantification of Emergence Delirium

It is difficult to interpret behavior in young children who cannot verbalize pain, anxiety, hunger, or thirst during awakening. The opinions of experienced clinicians are diverse on the point at which emergence extends to beyond "normal" [37]. Several rating scales [8,38] and visual analog scales that measure agitation have been used to measure EA in young children [12]. These scales, which may not be specific to ED, include behaviors like crying, agitation, and a lack of cooperation. However, they are problematic because they have not been psychometrically tested [8]. They have also been criticized as they predominantly assess psychomotor agitation.

Agitation, which is simple to assess, is frequently used as a descriptor for emergence behavior in children [11,32,36]. However, emotional distress and agitation are associated features rather than core features of a true delirium [39]. The behaviors measured by these scales overlap with the behaviors measured in validated behavioral pain assessment scales, such as the Face, Legs, Activity, Cry and Consolability (FLACC) scale, Children's and Infants' Postoperative Pain Scale (CHIPPS), or the Children's Hospital of Eastern Ontario Pain Scale (CHEOPS) [9].They may characterize children who are in pain or who are frightened or angry during emergence from general anesthesia rather than presenting with ED [3,9].

An accurate differentiation of delirium from other sources of agitation requires the identification of more complex symptoms of an acute mental disturbance. ED should not be diagnosed solely on the basis of crying and inconsolability [9]. Scales that diagnose ED on the basis of crying or inconsolability (Cravero, Watcha, or Cohen) may result in a high false-positive rate. The limitation of these scales may preclude comparisons among clinical trials, but more importantly it raises serious questions regarding measurement error and its reliability, as well as the validity of the research results [11,40].

Przybylo and colleagues [33] described an assessment tool that is based on the items listed in the Diagnostic and Statistical Manual of Mental Disorders, Fourth Edition (DSM-IV) for the diagnosis of delirium [39], but eliminated signs and symptoms that required verbalization or skill demonstration.

Sikich and Lerman [8] developed the PAED rating scale to produce a reliable and valid measurement tool for ED assessment without confounding variables such as pain. The PAED scale is a reliable tool to measure ED and involves five items: eye contact, purposeful actions, awareness of the surroundings, restlessness, and inconsolability (Table 16.1). According to the DSM-IV, three of these items are an important part of delirium and may be crucial to its differentiation from pain [39].

The first item of the PAED scale, "The child makes eye contact with the caregiver," and the third item of the scale, "The child is aware of his/her surroundings," reflect disturbances in the child's consciousness. "The child's actions are purposeful," addresses changes in the child's cognition during an ED reaction [8]. Children with ED are significantly more likely to display nonpurposefulness, averted, staring, or closed eyes, and nonresponsiveness. These behaviors were not significantly associated with pain and are believed to reflect the DSM-IV/5 diagnostic criteria for

Table 16.1 The Pediatric Anesthesia Emergence Delirium rating scale

	Not at all	Just a little	Quite a bit	Very much	Extremely
The child makes eye contact with the caregiver	4	3	2	1	0
The child's actions are purposeful	4	3	2	1	0
The child is aware of his/her surroundings	4	3	2	1	0
The child is restless	0	1	2	3	4
The child is inconsolable	0	1	2	3	4

delirium [9]. Restlessness and inconsolable crying reflect disturbance in psychomotor behavior and emotion, although they may also suggest pain or apprehension. The PAED scale score correlated negatively with the child's age and time to awakening and was significantly greater in children who received sevoflurane than in those who received halothane. The sensitivity of the scale is fair, although the true-positive rate (sensitivity) was 0.64, and the false-positive rate (1-specificity) was 0.14 [8].

Despite the reported high reliability, high validity, and applicability to young and alternate populations, the PAED scale still has some limitations. While the individual items have objective criteria, the score for each item is open to subjectivity thus raising a question about the scale's high inter-rater reliability [41].

It is possible that the scale items "The child is restless" and "The child is inconsolable" may reflect pain as well as ED. These items can be mistaken with symptoms of pain, tantrums, hunger, or distress. High scores on these items along with low scores on the other items produce a score within an ED classification [41]. Finally, there is no consensus regarding an appropriate cutoff score for the scale. Sikich and Lerman reported a sensitivity of 0.64 and a specificity of 0.86 with high (0.84) inter-observer reliability for a PAED score ≥ 10 points, which is the cutoff for an ED definition. Bajwa and colleagues stated that a PAED score ≥ 12 provides a sensitivity of 100% and a specificity of 94.5% using the evaluation of an expert anesthesiologist as the gold standard [38]. However, results of studies that rely on the clinical opinion of one observer, rather than a diagnostic tool to operationalize ED should be interpreted with caution. The variability of clinical opinions regarding normal and abnormal emergence may explain the different definitions of ED reported in the literature. Diagnosis of delirium in young children is complicated not only by developmental variability in the clinical presentations but also by the lack of a "gold standard" for ED [8,42].

Recently, Locatelli and colleagues [43] calculated a delirium-specific score (ED I) using the first three items of the PAED score (eye contact, purposeful actions, awareness of the surroundings) and a nonspecific delirium score (ED II) from the last two items on the PAED score (restlessness and inconsolability) to test the hypothesis that some items of the PAED scale may better reflect clinical ED than others. ED I was defined as a total of nine points or higher for the sum of the first three items of the PAED scale. ED II was recorded when the total value exceeded five points or higher on the last two items of the PAED scale. A delirium-specific score (ED I) of nine points or higher was highly correlated with ED in children with an effective caudal block for pain prevention. As ED I scores decreased with time, the signs of clinical ED also decreased effectively, indicating ED cases (sensitivity 93%) and non-ED cases (specificity 94%). In contrast, the last two items of the PAED scale (restlessness and inconsolability) represented a low sensitivity for the diagnosis of ED and may reflect pain instead of ED. ED II correctly identified non-ED cases (specificity 95%), but was not reliable in identifying ED cases (sensitivity 34%) [43].

In another study published recently, Malarbi and colleagues sought to develop a more specific method to measure delirium, which was based on the standard diagnostic criteria for delirium. They found that children with ED were more likely to display nonpurposefulness and lack of eye contact [9].

16.4 Prevention and Treatment

16.4.1 Midazolam

ED has been shown to be associated with preoperative anxiety and to be prevented by parental presence. Based on this, midazolam, an anxiolytic agent widely used as premedication, may appear to be a logical candidate in preventing EA. However, the influence of midazolam on emergence behavior seems to be somewhat controversial. Lapin and colleagues [44] and Ko and colleagues [45] reported a reduction of agitation in premedicated children, whereas McGraw and Kendrick [46] observed no difference at emergence and an increased incidence of adverse postoperative behavior up to 4 weeks after surgery. Midazolam, given as either premedication 30 min before induction of anesthesia or after induction, does not have a prophylactic effect against EA [16].

16.4.2 Propofol

Propofol delays or modifies emergence and could decrease the incidence of EA. Propofol showed an overall protective effect against EA. Continuous administration and a bolus dose at the end of anesthesia were protective, whereas a bolus at induction was ineffective in preventing EA [5,6,16,26,30].

16.4.3 Alpha-2 Adrenergic Agonists

Malviya and colleagues found that 2 µg/kg intravenous clonidine administered after anesthesia induction significantly reduced the incidence of EA in young children, but was associated with postoperative sleepiness [47]. Other studies have shown the efficacy of clonidine through oral or intravenous routes in preventing the incidence of EA. However, in most studies, postoperative behavior was assessed with a pain scale instead of an ED tool. Globally, alpha-2 adrenergic agonists were found to be protective against EA independently of the route of administration (intravenous or caudal), the alpha-2 adrenergic agonist used (dexmedetomidine or clonidine), and concurrent preoperative analgesia (none, preoperative analgesia, and local or regional analgesia) [16,35,37,47].

16.4.4 Regional Anesthesia

Regional anesthesia is associated with effective pain prevention and may reduce the incidence of ED [48]. Weldon and colleagues suggested that adequate analgesia produced by a caudal block reduced the incidence of ED after sevoflurane anesthesia when compared with halothane anesthesia. They hypothesized that inadequate pain prevention could explain, in part, the differences on ED incidence after sevoflurane and halothane anesthesia [36].

Pain control using a caudal block was associated with a significant reduction of ED incidence in children undergoing inguinal hernia repair [49].

Fascia iliaca compartment block reduced not only the intensity of pain, but also the severity of ED measured with the PAED scores for children undergoing elective orthopedic surgery [50].

Topical administration of tetracaine or sub-Tenon injection of lidocaine significantly reduced the incidence of ED after ophthalmologic surgery [51].

16.4.5 Fentanyl

Fentanyl has been associated with significant prevention and reduction of EA together with high efficacy for perioperative analgesia [16]. Cohen and colleagues stated that a dose of 2.5 µg/kg of fentanyl prevents EA while ensuring the rapid recovery associated with desflurane anesthesia in children undergoing adenoidectomy. The same group showed that concurrent use of fentanyl at a dose of 2.5 µg/kg results in a low incidence of EA in children receiving desflurane or sevoflurane anesthesia [40]. Galinkin and colleagues administered a dose of 2 µg/kg intranasal fentanyl after induction with sevoflurane, which resulted in therapeutic serum levels of fentanyl and decreased agitation after an ear tube placement [10]. Furthermore, Cravero and colleagues found that the incidence and duration of EA in patients receiving sevoflurane without surgery significantly decreased with the addition of 1 µg/kg^{-1} fentanyl at least 10 min before the end of anesthesia, without changes in the time to reach a discharge criterion [52].

Hypothalamic neurons of the hypocretin/orexin system, which regulate arousal and maintenance of the "awake" state, are inhibited by opioids through direct action on the cell bodies and indirectly by reducing excitatory synaptic tones via a presynaptic mechanism. These data suggest that a low incidence of ED in patients treated with fentanyl may be related to the actions of opioids on the hypocretin/orexin system [53].

16.4.6 Melatonin

Melatonin is a methoxyindole synthesized from tryptophan and secreted principally by the pineal gland. It has an endogenous circadian rhythm of secretion induced by the suprachiasmatic nuclei of the hypothalamus that is entrained to the light/dark cycle [54]. Premedication with melatonin, 3 mg or 0.5 mg/kg, decreased postoperative agitation when compared to placebo and was as effective as dexmedetomidine and midazolam [55]. Samarkandi and colleagues [56] found that melatonin (0.5 mg/kg) was associated with preoperative anxiolysis and sedation without impairment of cognitive and psychomotor skills or affecting the quality of recovery. Melatonin was as effective as midazolam in alleviating preoperative anxiety in children and was also associated with a tendency toward faster recovery and a lower incidence of postoperative excitement. Kain and colleagues [57] determined that the anxiolysis associated with 0.05, 0.2, or 0.4 mg/kg oral melatonin differed from that of midazolam in children scheduled for surgery. In contrast with previous results, they suggested that oral midazolam is a more effective anxiolytic than oral melatonin.

16.5 Decision-Making

Behavioral signs of ED often mimic those of postoperative pain during the first minutes after awakening. Whether the child is experiencing postoperative pain or ED or both, PACU nurses must lead the child safely through anesthesia recovery. The lack of distinctive distress behaviors that are unique to each of these conditions complicates the PACU nurses ability to assess and differentiate one condition from another. This may interfere with providing optimal treatment leading to a pharmacological treatment of a self-limiting disturbance (ED) or to a delayed treatment of postoperative pain.

A major confounding problem is determining whether inadequate pain relief or apprehensions are the cause of inconsolable crying. Obtaining a self-report of pain intensity is impossible in children experiencing delirium. Children who are disorientated and combative are unable to subjectively rate their pain.

Observation of behaviors may be used to assess both pain and ED. However, behavioral pain scores may be less reliable in children who are experiencing ED than in those who are experiencing pain only. Unfortunately, none of the behavioral scales that have been validated for assessing pain in children in the PACU have been tested for differentiating pain from ED. In our clinical practice we use the following steps.

16.5.1 Prevention of Emergence Delirium

We use anesthesia strategies that may reduce ED including: premedication with oral clonidine (instead of midazolam); pain prevention with local anesthetics or fentanyl; anesthesia maintenance with propofol (instead of sevoflurane or desflurane anesthesia).

16.5.2 Differentiating Pain from Emergence Delirium in the Postanesthesia Care Unit

Nonpurposeful activity, averted eyes or staring, and nonresponsiveness are all behaviors not significantly associated with pain and may reflect delirium. It is possible that children who demonstrate ED may transition into pain or other unsettled behavior. When applying the PAED scale, if a child does not "make eye contact with the caregiver," or is "unaware of his/her surroundings," and has "nonpurposeful actions" there is a high probability that they have ED. If the child is inconsolable and restless and presents low scores on other items (eye contact, purposeful actions, and awareness of the surroundings) they may have pain rather than ED.

16.5.3 Treatment

If we have doubts about the origin of distressing behaviors (pain or ED), we titrate fentanyl (0.5–1 μg/kg) to relieve the pain and distress associated with anesthesia and surgery. If the child presents a dangerous hyperactive motor behavior that requires constant restraint, a small bolus of propofol (0.5–1 mg/kg) is used.

References

1. Smessaert A, Schehr CA, Artusio JF Jr (1960) Observations in the immediate postanaesthesia period. II. Mode of recovery. British journal of anaesthesia 32:181-185
2. Eckenhoff JE, Kneale DH, Dripps RD (1961) The incidence and etiology of postanesthetic excitment. A clinical survey. Anesthesiology 22:667-673
3. Vlajkovic GP, Sindjelic RP (2007) Emergence delirium in children: many questions, few answers. Anesthesia and analgesia 104(1):84-91
4. Holzki J, Kretz FJ (1999) Changing aspects of sevoflurane in paediatric anaesthesia: 1975-99. Paediatric anaesthesia 9(4):283-286
5. Uezono S, Goto T, Terui K et al (2000) Emergence agitation after sevoflurane versus propofol in pediatric patients. Anesthesia and analgesia 91(3):563-566
6. Kol IO, Egilmez H, Kaygusuz K et al (2008) Open-label, prospective, randomized comparison of propofol and sevoflurane for laryngeal mask anesthesia for magnetic resonance imaging in pediatric patients. Clinical therapeutics 30(1):175-181
7. Smith HA, Fuchs DC, Pandharipande PP et al (2009) Delirium: an emerging frontier in the management of critically ill children. Critical care clinics 25(3):593-614
8. Sikich N, Lerman J (2004) Development and psychometric evaluation of the pediatric anesthesia emergence delirium scale. Anesthesiology 100(5):1138-1145
9. Malarbi S, Stargatt R, Howard K et al (2011) Characterizing the behavior of children emerging with delirium from general anesthesia. Paediatric anaesthesia 21(9):942-950
10. Galinkin JL, Fazi LM, Cuy RM et al (2000) Use of intranasal fentanyl in children undergoing myringotomy and tube placement during halothane and sevoflurane anesthesia. Anesthesiology 93(6):1378-1383
11. Cravero J, Surgenor S, Whalen K (2000) Emergence agitation in paediatric patients after sevoflurane anaesthesia and no surgery: a comparison with halothane. Paediatric anaesthesia 10(4):419-424
12. Beskow A, Westrin P (1999) Sevoflurane causes more postoperative agitation in children than does halothane. Acta anaesthesiologica Scandinavica 43(5):536-541
13. Cole JW, Murray DJ, McAllister JD et al (2002) Emergence behaviour in children: defining the incidence of excitement and agitation following anaesthesia. Paediatric anaesthesia 12(5):442-447
14. Voepel-Lewis T, Malviya S, Tait AR (2003) A prospective cohort study of emergence agitation in the pediatric postanesthesia care unit. Anesthesia and analgesia 96(6):1625-1630

15. Kain ZN, Caldwell-Andrews AA, Weinberg ME et al (2005) Sevoflurane versus halothane: postoperative maladaptive behavioral changes: a randomized, controlled trial. Anesthesiology 102(4):720-726

16. Dahmani S, Stany I, Brasher C et al (2010) Pharmacological prevention of sevoflurane- and desflurane-related emergence agitation in children: a meta-analysis of published studies. British journal of anaesthesia 104(2):216-223

17. Wells LT, Rasch DK (1999) Emergence "delirium" after sevoflurane anesthesia: a paranoid delusion? Anesthesia and analgesia 88(6):1308-1310

18. Faulk DJ, Twite MD, Zuk J et al (2010) Hypnotic depth and the incidence of emergence agitation and negative postoperative behavioral changes. Paediatric anaesthesia 20(1):72-81

19. Aouad MT, Nasr VG (2005) Emergence agitation in children: an update. Current opinion in anaesthesiology 18(6):614-619

20. Welborn LG, Hannallah RS, Norden JM et al (1996) Comparison of emergence and recovery characteristics of sevoflurane, desflurane, and halothane in pediatric ambulatory patients. Anesthesia and analgesia 83(5):917-920

21. Cohen IT, Finkel JC, Hannallah RS et al (2002) The effect of fentanyl on the emergence characteristics after desflurane or sevoflurane anesthesia in children. Anesthesia and analgesia 94(5):1178-1181

22. Demirbilek S, Togal T, Cicek M et al (2004) Effects of fentanyl on the incidence of emergence agitation in children receiving desflurane or sevoflurane anaesthesia. European journal of anaesthesiology 21(7):538-542

23. Valley RD, Freid EB, Bailey AG et al (2003) Tracheal extubation of deeply anesthetized pediatric patients: a comparison of desflurane and sevoflurane. Anesthesia and analgesia 96(5):1320-1324

24. Gupta A, Stierer T, Zuckerman R et al (2004) Comparison of recovery profile after ambulatory anesthesia with propofol, isoflurane, sevoflurane and desflurane: a systematic review. Anesthesia and analgesia 98(3):632-641, table of contents

25. Voepel-Lewis T, Burke C (2004) Differentiating pain and delirium is only part of assessing the agitated child. Journal of perianesthesia nursing: official journal of the American Society of PeriAnesthesia Nurses / American Society of PeriAnesthesia Nurses 19(5):298-299; author reply 9

26. Picard V, Dumont L, Pellegrini M (2000) Quality of recovery in children: sevoflurane versus propofol. Acta anaesthesiologica Scandinavica 44(3):307-310

27. Oh AY, Seo KS, Kim SD et al (2005) Delayed emergence process does not result in a lower incidence of emergence agitation after sevoflurane anesthesia in children. Acta anaesthesiologica Scandinavica 49(3):297-299

28. Pieters BJ, Penn E, Nicklaus P et al (2010) Emergence delirium and postoperative pain in children undergoing adenotonsillectomy: a comparison of propofol vs sevoflurane anesthesia. Paediatric anaesthesia 20(10):944-950

29. Konig MW, Varughese AM, Brennen KA et al (2009) Quality of recovery from two types of general anesthesia for ambulatory dental surgery in children: a double-blind, randomized trial. Paediatric anaesthesia 19(8):748-755

30. Aouad MT, Yazbeck-Karam VG, Nasr VG et al (2007) A single dose of propofol at the end of surgery for the prevention of emergence agitation in children undergoing strabismus surgery during sevoflurane anesthesia. Anesthesiology 107(5):733-738

31. Kain ZN, Caldwell-Andrews AA, Maranets I et al (2004) Preoperative anxiety and emergence delirium and postoperative maladaptive behaviors. Anesthesia and analgesia 99(6):1648-1654

32. Aono J, Ueda W, Mamiya K et al (1997) Greater incidence of delirium during recovery from sevoflurane anesthesia in preschool boys. Anesthesiology 87(6):1298-1300

33. Przybylo HJ, Martini DR, Mazurek AJ et al (2003) Assessing behaviour in children emerging from anaesthesia: can we apply psychiatric diagnostic techniques? Paediatric anaesthesia 13(7):609-616

34. Burke CN, Voepel-Lewis T, Hadden S et al (2009) Parental presence on emergence: effect on postanesthesia agitation and parent satisfaction. Journal of perianesthesia nursing: official journal of the American Society of PeriAnesthesia Nurses / American Society of Peri-Anesthesia Nurses 24(4):216-221

35. Bock M, Kunz P, Schreckenberger R et al (2002) Comparison of caudal and intravenous clonidine in the prevention of agitation after sevoflurane in children. British journal of anaesthesia 88(6):790-796

36. Weldon BC, Bell M, Craddock T (2004) The effect of caudal analgesia on emergence agitation in children after sevoflurane versus halothane anesthesia. Anesthesia and analgesia 98(2):321-326

37. Shukry M, Clyde MC, Kalarickal PL et al (2005) Does dexmedetomidine prevent emergence delirium in children after sevoflurane-based general anesthesia? Paediatric anaesthesia 15(12):1098-1104

38. Bajwa SA, Costi D, Cyna AM (2010) A comparison of emergence delirium scales following general anesthesia in children. Paediatric anaesthesia 20(8):704-711

39. (2000) American Psychiatric Association Task Force on, Dsm-IV Diagnostic and statistical manual of mental disorders: DSM-IV-TR: American Psychiatric Association

40. Cohen IT, Hannallah RS, Hummer KA (2001) The incidence of emergence agitation associated with desflurane anesthesia in children is reduced by fentanyl. Anesthesia and analgesia 93(1):88-91

41. Bong CL, Ng AS (2009) Evaluation of emergence delirium in Asian children using the Pediatric Anesthesia Emergence Delirium Scale. Paediatric anaesthesia 19(6):593-600

42. Scott GM, Gold JI (2006) Emergence delirium: a re-emerging interest. Seminars in Anesthesia 25(3):100-104

43. Locatelli BG, Ingelmo PM, Sahillio lu E et al (2012) Emergence delirium in children: a comparison of Sevoflurane and Desflurane anaesthesia using the PAED scale. Pediatric anesthesia. in press

44. Lapin SL, Auden SM, Goldsmith LJ et al (1999) Effects of sevoflurane anaesthesia on recovery in children: a comparison with halothane. Paediatric anaesthesia 9(4):299-304

45. Ko YP, Huang CJ, Hung YC et al (2001) Premedication with low-dose oral midazolam reduces the incidence and severity of emergence agitation in pediatric patients following sevoflurane anesthesia. Acta anaesthesiologica Sinica 39(4):169-177

46. McGraw T, Kendrick A (1998) Oral midazolam premedication and postoperative behaviour in children. Paediatric anaesthesia 8(2):117-1121

47. Malviya S, Voepel-Lewis T, Ramamurthi RJ et al (2006) Clonidine for the prevention of emergence agitation in young children: efficacy and recovery profile. Paediatric anaesthesia 16(5):554-559

48. Ghosh SM, Agarwala RB, Pandey M et al (2011) Efficacy of low-dose caudal clonidine in reduction of sevoflurane-induced agitation in children undergoing urogenital and lower limb surgery: a prospective randomised double-blind study. European journal of anaesthesiology 28(5):329-333

49. Araki H, Fujiwara Y, Shimada Y (2005) Effect of flumazenil on recovery from sevoflurane anesthesia in children premedicated with oral midazolam before undergoing herniorrhaphy with or without caudal analgesia. Journal of anesthesia 19(3):204-207

50. Kim HS, Kim CS, Kim SD et al (2011) Fascia iliaca compartment block reduces emergence agitation by providing effective analgesic properties in children. Journal of clinical anesthesia 23(2):119-123

51. Seo IS, Seong CR, Jung G et al (2012) The effect of sub-Tenon lidocaine injection on emergence agitation after general anaesthesia in paediatric strabismus surgery. European journal of anaesthesiology 29(1):53

52. Cravero JP, Beach M, Thyr B et al (2003) The effect of small dose fentanyl on the emergence characteristics of pediatric patients after sevoflurane anesthesia without surgery. Anesthesia and analgesia 97(2):364-367, table of contents

53. Li Y, van den Pol AN (2008) Mu-opioid receptor-mediated depression of the hypothalamic hypocretin/orexin arousal system. The Journal of neuroscience: the official journal of the Society for Neuroscience 28(11):2814-2819

54. Claustrat B, Brun J, Chazot G (2005) The basic physiology and pathophysiology of melatonin. Sleep medicine reviews 9(1):11-24

55. Isik B, Baygin O, Bodur H (2008) Premedication with melatonin vs midazolam in anxious children. Paediatric anaesthesia 18(7):635-641

56. Samarkandi A, Naguib M, Riad W et al (2005) Melatonin vs. midazolam premedication in children: a double-blind, placebo-controlled study. European journal of anaesthesiology 22(3):189-196

57. Kain ZN, MacLaren JE, Herrmann L et al (2009) Preoperative melatonin and its effects on induction and emergence in children undergoing anesthesia and surgery. Anesthesiology 111(1):44-49

Index

Printed in the United States
By Bookmasters